Endorsements

The book *Listen to Your Soul and Heal Your Body of Chronic Disease* is a personal journey of diagnosis, therapy, and self-healing. The book contains a great deal of material regarding body-soul attitudes, and advice on how to deal with a variety of diseases and how to achieve true recovery and health. The processes the author underwent are courageously detailed, and it is therefore certainly possible to learn from them regarding complicated questions such as what a disease is, why a disease breaks out at a particular time and harms one specific organ rather than another, what can be done to reach the root of a problem, what truly needs healing, and more. I recommend you read this slowly and internalize it.

Regards,

Dr. Chaim Rosenthal, *physician and homeopath, and head of the Israeli School of Homeopathy*

With startling directness and honesty, the author opens a window to her mental landscape, and to the inner demons and agonies that are present to a greater or lesser extent in almost every one of us.

The courage to open your eyes, face reality, and fearlessly

assume responsibility for your life, to shatter stereotypes and reexamine the "normal" versus the "abnormal," the possibility of making contact with the source of the pain—all these are central pillars in the ability to initiate change and spiritual healing and, the main point of the journey, to endlessly seek the connection that can accept and soothe the agonies of the soul.

You will find in this book much curiosity, human warmth, creativity and, most importantly, a reason to be hopeful.

Sigal Tzach, *psychotherapist and therapist of children and adults*

In her book *Listen to Your Soul and Heal Your Body of Chronic Disease*, Meirav Harel presents her incredible personal story, while navigating with down-to-earth language understandable to all readers through her personal travails to bring about her full healing from no fewer than seven physical, mental, and behavioral illnesses. As she progresses in the recovery process, she reaches deep spiritual insights that are the true basis of health.

Meirav presents to the reader, step-by-step, alongside the description of the real-life events she experienced, her holistic worldview and her faith in the existence of the physical, mental-emotional, energetic, and spiritual channels that are the basis of all diseases ("Disease is the physiological expression of the language of the soul" just as "the soul is the reflection of the spirit") and hence the ability to recover from the illness.

In this way, we can read about the critical importance of self-love and self-listening, the transition from rejection of responsibility to assuming responsibility and choice, the difference between the temporal-material and the eternal and enlightened, thankfulness, forgiveness, and more.

Instead of consciously creating illness, we can consciously create health.

We all need healing at the highest possible level through wholeness of body, spirit, and soul. The first step is understanding that it is possible. — Dr. Deepak Chopra

Dr. Amir Gilan, *family doctor, emergency physician, anesthesiologist, and anthroposophist*

Listen to Your Soul and Heal Your Body of Chronic Disease
Meirav Harel

Contact: meirav.harel1@gmail.com
Facebook: facebook.com/meirav.harel1

ISBN 978-1976175459

LISTEN TO YOUR SOUL AND **HEAL YOUR BODY** OF **CHRONIC DISEASE**

MEIRAV HAREL

*Dedicated to God, who gave me an opening,
and to my beloved Doron, who supported me*

Contents

PREFACE BY DR. AHARON ALEXANDROVITZ

Listen to Your Soul and Heal Your Body of Chronic Disease is a unique and important book in several respects. First of all, it is written by a woman who recovered from several illnesses, both physical and mental, which are usually incurable and require lifelong treatment.

Second, most therapeutic books concerning the link between the body and the soul were written by doctors, neglecting the patient's viewpoint, thoughts, feelings, and the entire process of the disease and recovery.

Third, this book touches upon a very crucial and controversial subject: the connection between the body, the soul, and the spirit. The medical community as a whole does not tend to recognize the great importance that the link between body and soul has to illness and diseases, in spite of many fine studies dealing with this link, and in spite of the important fact that between 20 percent and 40 percent of all diseases lack a defined medical diagnosis, or as they are called in the literature, "unexplained medical conditions." It is likely that most such diseases fall exactly into the seam between body and soul. Many studies point at the connection between the emotional state of the patient (and particularly stress) and disease and illness.

For many years now, the connection between a decline in lymphocyte activity (cells belonging to the immune system) and some studies indicate that cancer patients, when questioned a year before the outbreak of the disease, had statistically significantly elevated stress incidents. But one should also be cautious in assuming that a stressed individual is at increased risk of cancer.

Over the past few years, several studies have investigated the link between depression and recovery from myocardial infraction, and the unambiguous conclusion is that depression is the most significant known factor affecting recovery. Nonetheless, the medical community nearly ignores this link.

Beyond being a fascinating document of a journey of deep self-discovery with often painful expository revelations and exciting encounters with therapists and healers of various types, the book provides practical tools and recommendations on how to begin to find within yourself the unique method of healing that is right for you. In this sense, it is a novel book and offers a groundbreaking approach to self-healing.

Nonetheless, this book poses a challenge both to the patients and to their caregivers, including their doctors. For the patients, the challenge is to accept the fact that their diseases are expressions, primarily subconscious, of deep emotional distress with events either in the present or the past. Second, it is necessary to go on a long and often exhausting search for relevant caregivers in terms of who to approach and who to turn to for assistance. Finally, they must take into account that the journey they are embarking on is filled with ups and down and might take years, so they must gird themselves with considerable patience.

For caregivers and physicians, the challenge is first to accept the fact that a considerable portion of the diseases and the physical symptoms have an emotional aspect. Second, and this is very difficult for us, we need to accept that there are certain diseases and phenomena for which we have no ready-made remedies using the toolkit our training has provided us with. The third difficulty, which stems from the second, is that we must learn about an entire world of healing that we had never heard about before.

The hardest challenge to meet, both for patients and caregivers, is the author's final conclusion: "Self-love is the key to healing, the key to happiness, the key to acceptance, the key to calm, and the key to connecting ourselves with our deepest essential essence."

Dr. Aharon Alexandrovitz,
internist, psychotherapist, and lecturer at the Tel Aviv University School of Medicine

INTRODUCTION BY DR. ARYEH AVNI

Listen to Your Soul and Heal Your Body of Chronic Disease is an interesting book. It is an important book. It is a book that was missing on the shelf of proper medicine books. The book demonstrates how the author, without any formal certificate of medical education hanging on her wall, reaches insights on paths of recovery from a variety of diseases she had experienced, recovery for which the doctors treating her failed to provide.

The author, a curious woman who is deeply connected to her gut instincts, was able to treat all of her medical problems and solve them through understanding the sources of the problems from which the illnesses grew. **The author succeeded, on more than one occasion, in places where the finest experts in the field failed medically, and not only failed but failed to understand their failure or display any embarrassment about it.**

This book is meant for anyone interested in medicine, in the roots of diseases, in healing. I believe that this book **can also serve as a study text for some of our young doctors**, those who are prepared to learn what no one taught them in medical school.

I would recommend adding this book to any medical library. If the doctors just read what is written in the book (no additional examinations required), they might raise their level of medical understanding by understanding the essence of diseases and their root causes, and learning about alternative ways to resolve them.

Unfortunately, most of the older doctors are a lost cause. No change can be expected from them. Some patience is required to wait out the passing of this generation, whose existence revolves around the "medicine book." The new generation of doctors will no doubt be different. Will the addition of this book to the mandatory reading lists of doctors occur soon? Don't make me laugh. The medical profession reacts to developments; it does not initiate them.

It is not the doctors who brought to Israel acupuncture, Chinese medicine, herbal remedies, naturopathy, homeopathy, and other alternate medical branches. It is the "commoners" who have brought these wonderful branches of medicine to the benefit of us all. The Minister of Health is still stuck in the dark ages. The medical school masters have yet to include the teaching of proper nutrition in the medical degree study program. Professional snobbery and acquired arrogance prevent most doctors from listening to the wisdom of anyone who has not grown up within the hallowed halls of the medical guild.

When I completed my medical studies in Jerusalem, I felt that I was a member of the elite who knew all there was to know about healing. I didn't realize that the best experts in Hadassah (or the world) had ever cured a psoriasis patient, a blood pressure patient, a diabetes patient, an asthma patient (and so forth and so on, in regard to all chronic conditions). I needed a good smack to my head to change my mode of thought and see what proper medicine really was.

Meirav, the author of this book, did not need any cranial shock to sober up. She suffered from medical conditions, and she managed, on her own, to get out of the sandpits of medical pathology in which she found herself. And all that doctors proved with their prescriptions, as aforementioned, was their lack of understanding for the illness or for the healing process required.

I recall a case of a forty-nine-year-old woman (unmarried but living with her boyfriend) who arrived several years ago in my clinic. She had suffered from asthma from age ten onward. Her life revolved around inhalers from the steroid families and associated pills and injections. Her father was a world-renowned astrophysicist who lacked proficiency in Hebrew. She was examined by the best doctors in the world, but nothing helped alleviate her condition.

When she contacted me, I tried to reach the root of the problem. She did not have common asthma. Her difficulty, her sensation of suffocation, was concentrated inhalation. I interrogated her like a murder case coroner, from every possible angle. The root of the problem was sexual abuse by her father. He beat and strangled her, choked and raped her. Both her and her sister.

When the secret was exposed during the interrogation, the woman broke out in tears. The way to recovery had opened up. More talk, hugs, and tears were required to complete the recovery—not pills and inhalers. What manner of fool had prescribed all these injections, pills, and inhalers to her as a child, as a girl, as a woman? A terrible trauma was the cause of her pathology, which was misdiagnosed as a disease and "treated" accordingly. A multiparticipant display of ignorance, the ignorance of doctors who treated a false disease that could not be cured because it never existed to begin with.

The book *Listen to Your Soul and Heal Your Body of Chronic Disease* is the summary of the personal story of the author. This story includes a deep investigation of the problems she developed. The medical guild of doctors had no cure to offer her. Conventional medicine failed her, failed big-time. It was Meirav who cured herself.

The doctors will no doubt claim that medical miracles were involved. But there are no miracles in medicine. Miracles appear when the correct approach to healing is taken. The body yearns to be healthy. It sometimes needs the proper path to health to be marked out for it, but recovery is no miracle.

This book teaches us that if one path fails to provide a remedy, another path must be sought out. And I say that the all-too-common, all-too-available, all-too-conventional path of the various prescriptions is a multiyear failure.

A chronicle of blindness and ignorance, buttressed by arrogance.

I have no doubt that this book is an absolutely essential addition to the library of anyone who wishes to cure his body or his soul, and anyone who is willing to reach out to another patient who wants to struggle out of the conventional swamp in which he is mired.

Dr. Aryeh Avni,

graduate of Hadassah, Jerusalem, surgeon and gastroenterologist in his medical profession, graduate of homeopathy from Bar-Ilan University, author of A Romance with Nature: A Popular Guide for Homeopathic Medicine, The Milk Whips, Milk: Udder Nonsense, The Story of One Woman, What a Real Princess Eats, The Old Man and the Pretzels

Visit him at www.avni-med.com

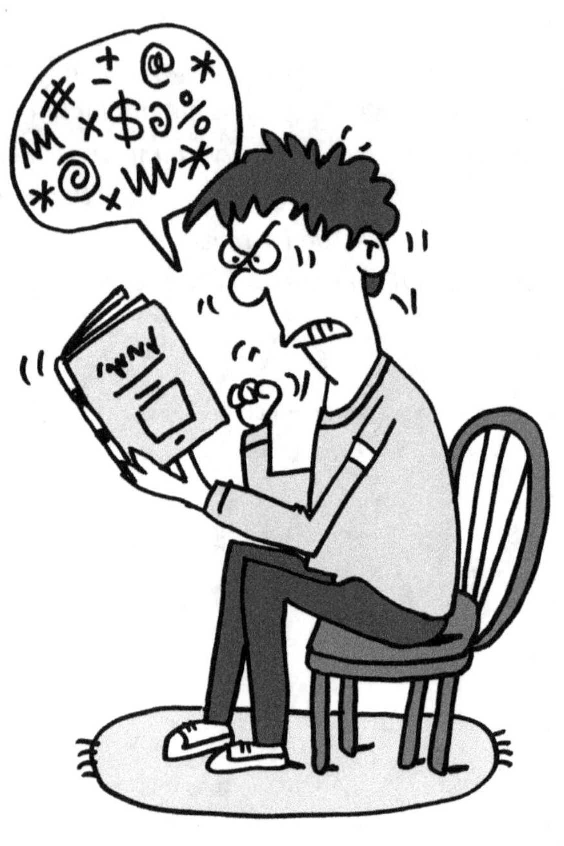

This book may well irritate many of you.

INTRODUCTION

I cured myself from chronic diseases and pains, and here I will tell you how.

This book has the potential to aggravate and piss off many of you, and for that I apologize in advance. It will touch your bare nerves, challenge your thinking, shatter many a well-cherished belief and paradigm, kick your sacred cows, and lead you to blurt out, "What a crock!" or "What utter nonsense!" out loud, so everyone can hear you.

In order to cure ourselves from diseases, we must agree to accept, without argumentation, a number of uncommon and unconventional truths that some will call deluded. These include:

- Something deep within us created our disease, without our knowledge and without asking us.
- The responsibility for our disease lies with us.
- We have the power to decide whether we recover from the disease or continue to suffer from it.

If these three sentences choked a guffaw out of you, I invite you to close the book for now, place it back on the bookshelf or return it to whomever gave it to you, and continue to live your life with the disease and with the pills. It's all right, not everyone needs to be healthy, and not everyone needs to make a change. Hey, you're already used to living with the pain, and it isn't really that bad, and the doctor says there is nothing to be done, right? Maybe your time has not come yet, and that's fine. Really, it is!

The last thing I want to do is to annoy you and add to the burden the disease or pain you are afflicted with is imposing upon you, or to waste your valuable time. What I do want to do is help you. This book was written in order to help you. The obligatory question is: Do you want to help yourself? Another obligatory question is: Do you have the courage required to do so?

If the answer to both questions is affirmative, and if you accept the three aforementioned truths (or at least don't dismiss them out of hand, but maintain an open mind), then I invite you to join me on a short journey toward the beginning of the path that will lead you to self-healing, or at least lead you to doubt your disease and not accept it as a done deal for which the only remedy is more and more pills.

The other thing I want to do, which I view as no less important than the first, is to give you hope. To open up a hatch, even if it is no more than a tiny crack, to the belief that self-healing from diseases is possible. Why is it important for me to do this? Because nobody ever did that for me, not from my nearby environment. I had to build up this faith in myself on my own. It was a difficult and challenging process with many near-breaking points—and the process took years because there was no structure, no methodology I could follow or act upon—but at the end of the day, I did it. I made it.

Here is a list of my many diseases:

- Asthma: I was defined as asthmatic for eighteen years.
- Bulimia: I have been shoving fingers down my throat for eighteen years.
- Bipolar disorder: For over eight years, I oscillated between clinical depression and thrilling manias.
- Drug addiction: For twenty years, I smoked light drugs on a daily basis.
- I successfully overcame the chronic pains from two disc herniations and two back surgeries. I ached in my lower back for ten years.
- Migraines: My head pounded for eighteen years.
- In addition, I am still on a journey to heal my hypothyroidism, which has been malfunctioning since the year 1999.

So whether or not the above list impressed you, it is time to start believing that it is possible to heal yourself, because it is. We can heal ourselves from illness. It is possible to live without pills. Look at me—I did so on several occasions. And that was a pretty respectable collection of aches and pains, wouldn't you say?

I will tell you here how I started on this path and why, how I eventually succeeded, and what worked for me and what didn't, and give you some food for thought. In particular, you should leave aside what I tell you and feel what my words do to you, how they touch you, where they vibrate. You are invited to check out everything said here on your own on the University of the World Wide Web, which is open to everyone and, in spite of its size, is very pleasant and welcoming.

Try it. What do you have to lose? The pain? The misery? The pills? The suffering?

A happy and calm life to you all!

PART 1

BACKGROUND TO THE GUIDE

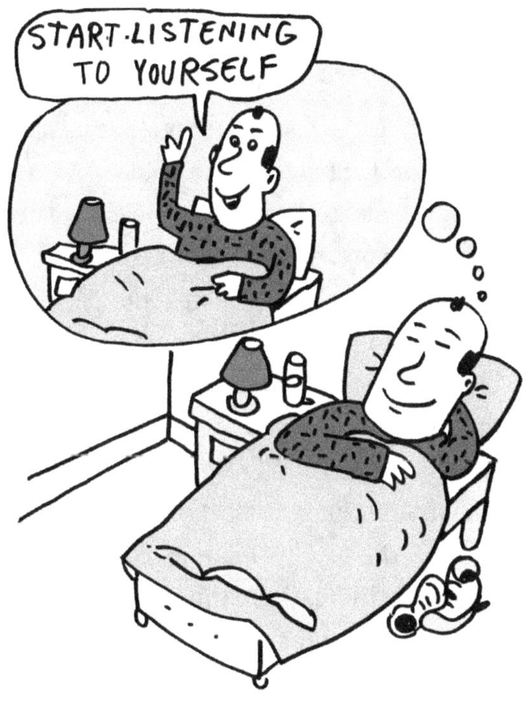

Our soul speaks to us in many languages:
our emotions, our sensations, our dreams, our
reflexive responses, and also our diseases.

CHAPTER 1
THE LANGUAGE OF THE SOUL

Our soul does not speak with words. It has no heart-rending monologues or stirring speeches that leave us breathless to share, because the language of the soul is not made up of words. Its language is not the linear speech we are familiar with, where any word spoken has a meaning, intention, or needs behind it, which enables the environment to understand us or our needs at that moment.

To be honest, the above sounds like a sad joke, given how the couches of psychotherapists all over the world are filled with people screaming that "No one is listening to me" or "No one understands me" or "I don't understand myself." But let us stay off the psychotherapist couch for now; there is plenty of time for that later in the book.

One word after another forms a sentence and then another sentence, and we have achieved some passing comprehension of the mechanism of speech.

How then does one—can one—communicate without words? How can we pass on messages to ourselves or to the environment without speech? Or tell a tale? Or give a speech? Or badger our unfortunate audience to exhaustion?

The soul has no single language. There is not a single way to pass on a message. The soul uses several different means of communication, choosing between them according to circumstances—depending on the time, environment, and situations where it is present, and on its own needs. (These include conscious needs such as the desire to be loved or to belong, and subconscious needs such as self-defense or, at a more primordial level, survival and existence).

Among the myriad languages of the soul are our emotions—what we feel at any given moment toward a given individual in a given situation. Are we angry? Are we happy? Are we hurt? Are we offended?

We can develop our awareness of these sensations. What do we feel at any given moment toward a given individual in a given situation? Excitement? Apathy? Fear? Confusion? Focus? Clarity? The experience is essentially physical with "mental overtones" here and there.

Dreams are also an inseparable part of the languages of the soul, playing many roles and fulfilling many functions. For the sake of this discussion, we will focus on the need of the soul to tell us a story, its own story. Our soul will use dreams to deliver a message to us, to remind us of things we had chosen to forget for one reason or another, to point us along a certain path, to guide us on the process we are undergoing, to explain our experiences. What is a recurring nightmare if not the cry of the soul: "Please pay attention to me! I will not let you forget me! Help me help us!"

This is where our automatic impulsive reactions can also be found—how we respond in a given moment toward a given individual in a given situation. These are our uncontrollable responses, those that simply occur automatically without being planned, or in many cases occur exactly the opposite of how we planned, wanted, or hoped for. For the most part, dear friends, this is our less attractive side. It is precisely the aspect of ourselves that we most want to conceal from others or ourselves that reveals itself in this automatic impulse.

Still, in order to avoid being negative and ruining your mood completely, let us also consider our positive automatic impulses, such as the impulse to aid someone in need. If we see a child about to be run over, and rush toward him, or see someone who collapses in the street quickly move to help, we do not stop ourselves to ask, "Hold on, should I offer him help? But I am hurrying to get to my meeting or catch my train or reach an incredible sale." We just do it, automatically, without thinking about it. This is a charming aspect all humans possess.

Of course, if we pass down the street a minute after this stranger had fallen and see that there are already people crowding around him, our automatic impulse might be: "Oh well, many people are already helping him, so he doesn't really need my help. They are doing fine without me. What can I contribute?" We will not feel bad about ourselves at that moment, and that is fine because we are hurrying to the important meeting, to the last train or to the incredible sale before all the great deals are grabbed off the shelf.

But there is another way for our souls to speak to us—through diseases and afflictions. **A disease, in and of itself, is a physiological expression of the language of the soul,**

like a signpost meant to mark out that a problem exists, that an incident is occurring that must be addressed. There is something here that must not be forgotten, even if we really want to forget it, or even forgot that we forgot it or are repressing it.

Many of these incidents involve physical, mental, or emotional pain, or an unresolved conflict, and our automatic tendency is to suppress this memory, deny it, and move on, because "What does not kill us makes stronger" and to hell with it, let's move on and put it behind us, we've survived and it's all over...isn't it? However, it is not really over, and we have not really moved on. Perhaps we think it is over, perhaps we have forgotten about it on the everyday level and have returned to our routine, but that is only an illusion, because the soul does not forget.

Even the physical body cannot forget, because the experiences we try to suppress reside in the memory of the body's cells, digging in with no defined exit date. And that, dear friends, to make a long story short, is the source of all our maladies and illnesses. To that basic cause, additional parameters (which will be discussed later) are added. But as of this point, that is enough.

The most important question we now need to ask ourselves is: Do we choose to listen to our souls? Do we choose to try to hear them and the stories they are trying to tell us? Because we do not really have to. Not as such. Nobody is pointing a gun at our temples and threatening us to "Listen to me or die." Not in day-to-day life anyway.

When is the gun pointed at our temple? When death is

staring us in the whites of our eyes in the form of a heart attack, a stroke, cancer, or any other terrible disease. Only then are we prepared to stop and listen, because we want to live. Very much so. However, on a day-to-day basis, in our routine, we have all learned how to live our lives with pains of one intensity or another or with various diseases at differing intensity levels.

At a certain age, pains begin in various locations of the body, and at that age or one not far removed, one begins to take pills for various diseases or pains, and one learns to live with it, because what is the alternative? Complaining? How would that help? Where would that get us? And besides, there is no choice and there is nothing to do about it anyway, and we have learned how to be happy with pains and with the diseases and the accompanying pills, because what do we have in this life if not our happiness, right?

Why Is It so Hard for Us to Listen to Our Soul?

We can spend an entire lifetime without listening to the soul. The question to be asked is: Do we want to listen to it? Will we want to listen to it now, when we know that it also speaks to us through disease and affliction? Will we want to hear the story it is longing to tell us? And if we do, will we choose to do something about it? Will we choose to change the situation?

For most people, listening to the soul is a difficult if not impossible task. That is a cruel and painful truth, but it is the truth, and we will win only by acknowledging it.

To me, there are three main reasons that explain why it is so difficult for us to listen to our soul, even though it is supposedly part of us, flesh of our flesh, blood of our blood. These three reasons are very simple to understand, but just as they are amazingly simple, so are they also incredibly hard to address. (Incidentally, this is something else that life taught me: The simpler a solution is in principle, the harder it is for people to implement. It is their very simplicity that impedes taking remedial action.)

It is this very simplicity that makes implementing the knowledge difficult. And so it is with the solution offered here for dealing with your ailments: Choose to listen to your soul. Painfully simple, is it not?

Why am I saying that the reasons easiest to understand are hardest to address? Because reality proves this is true. Why else would people not always implement these solutions? After all, we all want to be healthy, don't we? None of us likes suffering, right? (Let us put aside for a moment people who enjoy the attention that suffering nets them much more than they suffer from the pain.)

No one likes being limited or deprived by a physical disability, right? No one likes being dependent on pills, just like most people do not enjoy eating just healthy food, do they? But lo and behold, what is happening all around you—pains and ailments of all types and kinds, in spite of the super-advanced medicine at our service over the past generation. And it's not getting better, only worse. This is the time to remind you to keep an open mind, because here come the causes for our difficulty in listening to our soul.

The first reason is that in order to listen to our soul, we must first recognize that we are the creators of our own reality!

We created this disease in our life, and that, my friends, is quite a task for most people, or perhaps I should say for almost all people! What does it even mean to create a reality? Do you mean I wanted to suffer? Wanted to be hurt? Did I choose to be dependent on pills? I did not choose this, I did not create this—what kind of nonsense is this?

Well, here is the thing—we did create this. We create our own reality. That is what we all do here in this world, even if we are not aware of it, do not believe in it, or do not accept it. This process is incepted in the subconscious, our personality's hidden aspect, and is then established and supported in reality by the conscious, everyday aspect of our personality.

The second cause of our difficulties in listening to our soul is the additional step we must take in the form of taking responsibility! This disease is my responsibility and it is my responsibility to heal myself!

It is always good to have someone else to blame. My mother taught me this when I was just a child. Always look for someone else to blame for your situation because passing on the blame is always in your best interest! It is true, my mother said this lightheartedly when I fought with my sister and argued with her over this or that petty reason, but in truth this was not at all funny and one of the most important lessons I learned in life. She was completely right.

For most of us, it is difficult to impossible to take responsibility or accept the responsibility of our own words, deeds, and behavior. It is so much easier to blame others. Blaming the other comes naturally, feels better while we do it, and even makes us feel better about ourselves afterward. For the most part, we are not even aware that we are diverting responsibility for our own deeds and misdeeds to someone else, and it is precisely this lack of awareness that is the cause of our continued suffering from various diseases and maladies, or else makes us dependent on pills.

The third cause of our difficulty in listening to our soul is the most painful one: We do not want to feel the underlying cause of our hurt again.

We have put so much effort into fleeing from it, forgetting it, erasing it, coloring it with other colors from the pitch black that is its essence. So why go back there? No way. I'll just lay it out straight. Yes, it probably will hurt to pick at that emotional scar again, no matter what format the emotion takes—feeling insulted, discriminated, angry, jealous, sad, ashamed, or any one of the dozens of negative emotions we experience throughout our lives all too many times.

But is it not better to feel this pain again deliberately and temporarily after preparing for it, in order to exorcise it once and for all? Getting rid of it for ever and ever? Think about it for a moment. This is your pain; you known it better than I do. Think about hurting from it once again but for a final time, and then letting go.

I have two encouraging things to tell you at this stage:

1. The sense of satisfaction you will feel after you recuperate from your disease is worth all the suffering and temporary pain you will feel. It is guaranteed in advance that you will feel this satisfaction if you do indeed recover! This has been tried and proven in thousands of cases of people from all over the world who cured themselves of diseases. You will simply be healthy!

2. It does not really matter right now what is the thing, event, action, or trauma (one time or ongoing) you experienced in the past that is the source of your present suffering. Regardless, unlike the painful past, where whatever happened happened—likely without you choosing it or wanting it—now, at this point in time, you are exercising your free will and choosing to be there, choosing to feel once again the suffering or the pain but from a more mature, self-aware place that is more accepting and understanding, and that makes all the difference in the world. Dear friends, this difference means everything. It will hurt much less and it will be temporary. It will pass. Encouraging, isn't it?

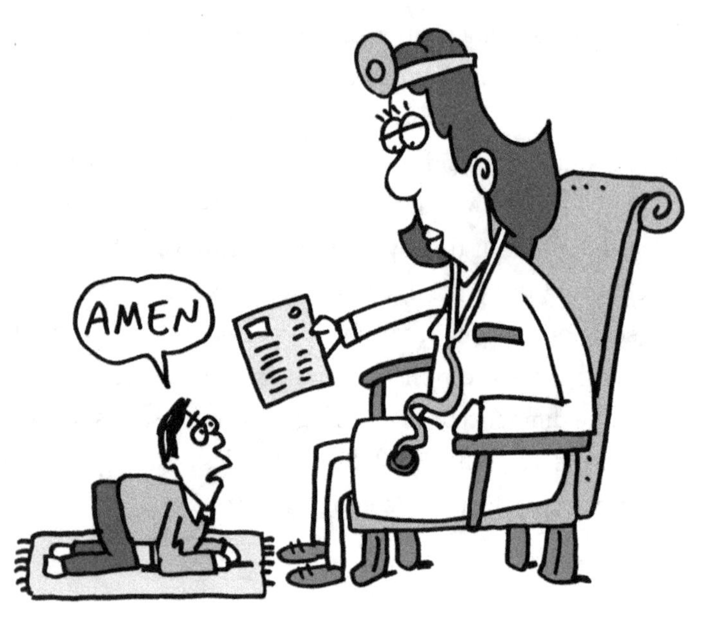

Most people have blind faith in doctors, as if God Himself had descended from on high to speak to them.

CHAPTER 2

MEDICAL INDOCTRINATION

I'll start with a confession: In addition to the three internal obstacles interfering with our ability to listen to our soul and heal ourselves, there is an additional, external obstacle. Running into this obstacle can be infuriating; it certainly infuriated me at the time!

What is this obstacle? It can be summed up as medical indoctrination. Whether we are aware of it or consciously accept its premises, everyone who grew up in a Western society has been exposed to, and subconsciously molded by, this indoctrination—both patients and physicians. What are the premises of this omnipresent indoctrination?

- The business of modern medicine is to cure all diseases, chronic as well as acute.
- Physicians know everything there is to know about illness and health.
- It's all in your genes.

Am I speaking about the ill-informed medical conventions of previous generations, or the imperfect practice in developing countries? No, everything in this chapter refers to modern, twenty-first century Western medicine. This advanced, high-technology, scientifically and experimentally based discipline is making quantum leaps forward in certain fields—even as it remains mired in the past in the most important field of all, helping us be healthy.

So why is this medical indoctrination making it hard for us to listen to our souls and cure ourselves? Because it is an insanely impenetrable obstacle. Because it is an essential part of how modern health systems operate worldwide, and because the bottom line it keeps on pushing at us is that the way to deal with disease, any disease, is to take our patented drugs once, twice, or three times a day.

Yes, you will be told, you run off to your shrink and sob about how you weren't hugged enough as a child. Sure, they will tell you to eat more vegetables and less red meat or dairy products, and don't forget to exercise. It can't hurt, but it also won't cure your chronic disease or high blood pressure or cancer. For that, you need your pills. That's just the way it is, and there is no alternative. So let's all be good, indoctrinated little boys and girls, smile, and wash them down with a glass of water, shall we?

The premises of this indoctrination, on which I will expand below, slay any hope for self-healing before it can even be born. And if there is no hope, why should we even make the effort necessary to succeed?

PREMISE #1: THE BUSINESS OF MODERN MEDICINE IS TO CURE ALL DISEASES, CHRONIC AS WELL AS ACUTE.

"We have not lost faith, but we have transferred it from God to the medical profession."

— George Bernard Shaw

I'll start with the punchline: The business of modern medicine, as far as chronic diseases are concerned, is not to cure the disease and make the patient healthy. Instead, it is to suppress its symptoms with periodic doses of patented medication.

Medical students do not learn about health and how to generate and maintain it; all they learn about is diseases and the drugs that should be used to treat them. It is the disease which is the focus of treatment, and the overall, long-term well-being of the patient is often overlooked.

There is nothing groundbreaking in this declaration. Many voices, both from within the medical system itself and from without it have spoken about the fallacies of how the medical system treats chronic diseases. But what is the underlying cause for this pathology of medical practice? The problem is that medical **systems worldwide, and medical schools as an inseparable part of these systems, are dependent on the pharmaceutical companies. Many of them are even funded, to a greater or lesser extent, openly or discreetly, by them.**

If you stop to think about it, it all makes perfect sense. The pharmaceutical companies are massive corporations whose stocks are traded in Wall Street and various stock exchanges worldwide. Economics 101 teaches that if a company wishes to survive, it must turn a maximal profit above all else, for they are accountable to stockowners.

So take a guess—how can the average multinational pharmaceutical company ensure its ongoing survival and prosperity? That's right, by ensuring that billions of people remain dependent on the drugs it produces. Trafficking in diseases suddenly seems like a good business plan, doesn't it? The pharmaceutical companies are businesses that turn a profit when we are ill and lose money when we are healthy.

The reason we patients don't wise up to this is that we are so brainwashed that we cannot internalize this basic fact, that the pharmaceutical companies cannot afford to allow themselves to want us to be healthy. If we stopped taking their drugs, what would be left for them to do? How would they make a living?

But, you may well say, doctors do want us to be healthy. Well, that is true enough. They do honestly want us to get better. Nobody puts himself through medical school and the hellish shifts that follow in order to become a drug peddler. They do it because they generally desire to help people. Unfortunately, they have never been taught about how to help ill patients return to health and live independently of symptom-suppressing pills.

How do I know this? Well, for one thing, I've listened to hundreds of physicians who worked within the system confess exactly this. These physicians studied for many years and practiced medicine for many more, yet they have never been able to permanently cure, nor temporarily suppress, the symptoms of patients suffering from chronic diseases. They simply couldn't restore their patients to a healthy and balanced condition, because they were forced to use the wrong tools for the job. These physicians had the courage to say publicly what many more medical practitioners continue to agree with silently. Dozens of them wrote books diagnosing how the medical profession failed their patients.

What all of them had been taught in their long, long, long time in medical school, residency, and specialization studies is about diseases and their symptoms, and the drugs relevant to these diseases and symptoms. And once they had completed their official studies, they continued to keep up-to-date on the latest medical articles, because medical technology and practice is always evolving.

Take a guess—what did all of these articles talk about? That's right, new drugs, based on the most up-to-date scientific studies. Do you need to put any effort into guessing who funds these studies? Who are the only players who have the money to fund these studies?

I invite you to YouTube to watch the testimonies of whistleblowers who have worked in the pharmaceutical industry and who had the courage to speak out and reveal how things happen behind closed doors. You will hear horror stories about side effect reports that were silenced or shredded, and how batches of medications that killed and/or paralyzed and/or triggered new diseases left the shelves quietly without any party being held accountable or punished for it.

Later, I will share my personal experience with such

a scandal. None of this is new. On the contrary—all this is information that has been available for far too long without any fundamental response or change of behavior by the medical profession or by us, their patients.

So what can you do about it? Not much more than being aware. Awareness of the medical indoctrination and its falsehoods and partial truths is the first step toward taking personal responsibility for your health.

Take-home message: The role of prescription drugs is not to cure diseases. The reason they were created is to change or ablate certain physiological or biochemical processes in the body in order to suppress certain symptoms.

PREMISE #2: PHYSICIANS KNOW EVERYTHING THERE IS TO KNOW ABOUT ILLNESS AND HEALTH.

Physicians do not know everything. They know a lot. Their brains are crammed with entire libraries of medical text-books, scientific journals, and years of experience in treating patients in the ways they have been taught. That cannot be disputed. But still, they don't know everything.

How do I know that? Because many medical practitioners worldwide are brave enough, desperate enough, or frustrated enough with the status quo to violate the informal taboo of the medical profession and share the limits of their knowledge and the vast vistas of their ignorance about all matters related to curing people and making them healthy again. They do so through documentaries, books they have written, and lectures given worldwide.

The use of a well-balanced diet as a means to affect overall health is a subject that is not included in the curricula of modern medical schools. The rare nutrition class does not emphasize the multiparameter healthy lifestyle or its critical importance to overall health. In addition, many of the supposedly educational materials about nutrition topics used in those rare lessons are funded by the dairy and meat industries. And this is a worldwide phenomenon.

The result is ignorance by medical practitioners in regard to all things related to nutrition and a healthy lifestyle. Yes, ignorance is a harsh word, but that is what physicians who were educated within the system testify regarding their shortcomings upon graduation. I am merely relaying their own conclusions.

Correct nutrition as a means of influencing health is not even included in the hospitals themselves! If any of you have had the dubious pleasure of being hospitalized or visiting hospitalized loved ones, you can easily see that the hospital menu is far from providing a diet good for patients and their immune systems. What the food served to patients should do is literally bombard their immune systems with vitamins and minerals, strengthening and supporting them in fulfilling their role. This issue is critical, particularly for patients struggling for their lives.

In practice, the hospital menu is reflective of various economic considerations that are irrelevant to the patient's well-being, and no one tells the patients how important it is to support their immune systems with proper nutrition, particularly when they are fighting infections or tumors, and that this is even more critical if their immune systems are being bombarded with toxins that are weakening them.

Studies concentrating on reviews and conclusions of thousands of cases of "spontaneous healing" (and not just from cancer), even those published in the most prestigious medical journals, are also excluded from the curriculum of modern medical schools. No one in the system ever stopped and said, "Hold on, perhaps we should devote 5 percent or so of our vast curricula to studying these cases, to studying the common elements in the thousands of stories of former patients."

Many of those patients had already been given up as lost causes by modern medicine and had been instructed to make peace with their death and to bid farewell to their family and loved ones. And yet, they are still among us, healthy and drug-free. True, these cases are the exceptions, not the rule, but the systemic decision to disregard these cases and exclude them from the body of knowledge on which physicians are trained produces physicians who know a great deal about diseases, but not enough about health and self-healing.

So why is the knowledge of physicians so limited in certain respects? Their limitations are not determined by some objective limit on the knowledge that the human brain can hold, **but because physicians only know what the pharmaceutical industries train them to know.** The entire health system and its myriad limitations and defects are rigged to transform them, over many years, however they might feel about it, into "disease technicians."

This term disease technicians is one that physicians themselves use to describe their predicament. A touching, reliable, and honest disclosure of this predicament can be found in Dr. Bernie S. Siegel's book *Love, Medicine and Miracles: Lessons Learned about Self-Healing from a Surgeon's Experience with Exceptional Patients*. Dr. Jerome Groopman also touches upon it in his book *How Doctors Think*.

Doctors learn so much about diseases and infections, but no one teaches them to ask one simple question: "Why?" Why has the disease shown up to begin with? What is its cause? What are the environmental or mental or physical conditions that enable it to erupt? Why does the infection, or the bacterium, or the virus attack one person and not another, even if both are present in the same space and exposed to the exact same microbes? What characteristics does the infected person possess that form the petri dish upon which it all evolved?

Physicians work in a hectic system and do not have time to ask these questions, let alone find the answers to them. But we will touch further upon those constraints in the next chapter when we enter the doctors' minds.

Why is this indoctrination? Because most people possess blind faith in their physicians, and feel during their medical visitations as if God Himself had descended from the heavens and pronounced their fate, which is why whatever the doctor pronounces does, in fact, happen to most people.

If a person is certain that his physician is 100 percent correct, even if in practice his diagnosis might be mistaken, he will not be able to help himself. He will not be capable of skepticism, of wondering whether perhaps there is some other cause or solution for his problem; nor will he consider whether there is any advantage for a novice who had not studied for many years in dealing with his particular issues. After all, a person who has not studied conventional medicine for many years is much more open to new ideas, and does not rule anything out, because he has nothing to lose besides his own life and health.

PREMISE #3: IT IS ALL IN YOUR GENES.

One of the greatest surprises in my journey toward self-healing was the discovery that our lives are not truly controlled by our genes. Genetics is not really responsible for whether a disease afflicts us. It turns out that genes control nothing and that they cannot turn themselves off or on. They merely respond to stimuli and signals from the environment. That environment can be our nutrition or our thoughts and beliefs, or all of them together. Amazing, isn't it? (Excellent sources for the study of this subject are the books *Anticancer* by Dr. David Servan-Schreiber and *The Biology of Belief* by Dr. Bruce Lipton. Each references dozens of scientific studies supporting these assertions.)

So what are the implications of this wrong premise? Well, for one, if you have been told for your entire life that everyone in your family dies from a heart disease at the age of forty-five, then guess what? You are likely to be headed in that direction at the age of forty, even if you happen to be adopted.

If you have heard, ever since you became a woman, that the family history is filled with women who died of breast cancer at an early age, take a moment to consider how that knowledge alone may have increased your chances to develop that condition. Could your belief or fear have triggered the latent gene?

If a doctor tells a man that he has a hereditary disease, to what extent did the patient's tendency to view any pronouncement by his physician as being as authoritative as the word of God impact his ability to summon the willpower required to take responsibility, and control, of his own health? To what extent would it affect his chances of recovery?

So why is this indoctrination false? Because it has been scientifically proven many years ago that **genetics is no more than a potential whose realization is subject to our own emotional interpretation and to the environmental and nutritional conditions we are exposed to. And yet, many diseases are transmitted from generation to generation not due to "bad genes" but due to false beliefs about the disease and in general that are imprinted in us from childhood**. If a person is sure that this is the truth and the whole truth, then why should he be mindful when he is told he can cure himself from the disease?

My psychiatrist repeatedly told me over many years that the chemical imbalance in my mind responsible for the bipolar disorder from which I suffer was genetic and hereditary, that it could not be cured, and that I would have to balance it, until the end of my life, with various prescription drugs. The simple fact that no one in my family suffers, or had ever suffered from, a similar mental condition was irrelevant to the genetically predetermined fate he pronounced upon me. As far as he was concerned, the existence of this condition in my family tree was a fact I was unaware of or a buried family secret, because my condition fit the indicators his textbooks taught him to classify as genetic.

For many years, I believed him that it was hereditary. So the professor said, and one does not argue with either one's doctor or one's genes. (I will expand upon my eventual closure with this psychiatrist in chapter 10.)

There is another potentially infuriating point I wish to make concerning genetics, so take a deep breath and brace for impact. **The moment we blame our genes for what ails us, we abandon any responsibility for improving our condition. Blaming your genes means that you are blaming someone or something external and not taking responsibility for that issue.**

To demonstrate with the most obvious example, when people say that a certain family has a genetic tendency for obesity, they are ignoring the fact that the only thing that definitely and unambiguously contributes to obesity in a given family is the tendency of the family members to overeat. This overindulgence probably stems from an absence of self-acceptance or love of oneself, and is sometimes a defense mechanism. There are many, many reasons for overeating and/or emotional eating, but genetics is not one of them, and **it is time to stop blaming your genes for everything**.

I will touch on emotional eating later on, from my

perspective as an ex-bulimic, and will detail specifically what helped me get over my bulimia and restore health, balance, and love of self, resolving the root cause of my disorder.

For now, it is sufficient to sum up the issue of not taking responsibility for our health by saying that if a child is obese, this is not necessarily a sign of a genetic predisposition to obesity, but rather a sign that his parents did not instill in him knowledge of proper nutrition or good eating habits, or give him a personal example in this regard. I have no intention to be judgmental of these hypothetical parents or anyone else; I just want to emphasize that there is no point in blaming the genes. Doing so simply obstructs listening to the story our soul is trying to tell us through (in this case) eating disorders and obesity.

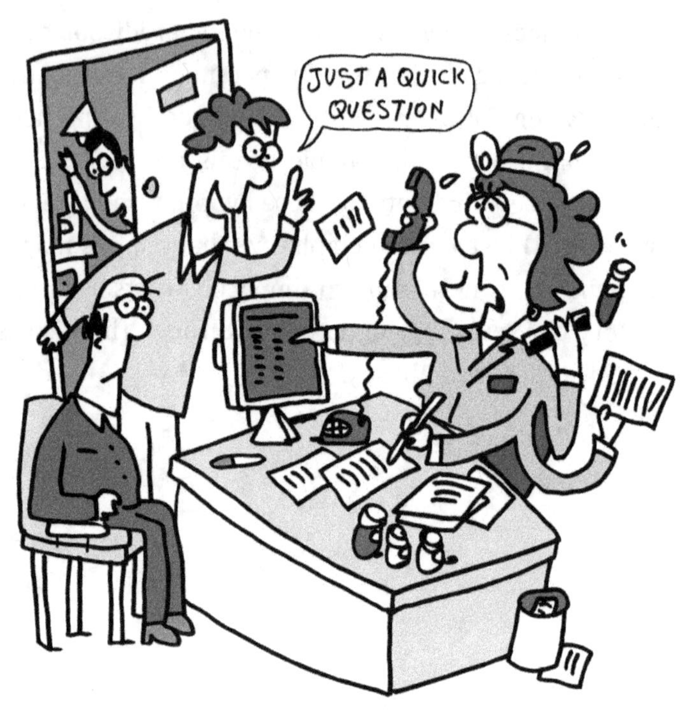

Doctors work very hard within a system that is insensitive to their needs and driven by the profit motive.

CHAPTER 3

A VOYAGE IN THE MIND OF A DOCTOR

Proper disclosure: Becoming a doctor was my childhood dream. When I grew up, I understood that this was mostly my father's dream, and I was a classic example of an older daughter striving to please her daddy. Still, I enjoyed my expanded biology studies in high school and everything involving our farm animals. My love for the magic of life in general, and the human body in particular, led me to become a medic during my military service (which is obligatory in Israel for anyone between the ages of eighteen and twenty), and to fly to Italy to undergo a six-month preparatory program for medical studies.

Within that framework, I studied chemistry, physics, biology, and mathematics—all in Italian. I wanted to fulfill my dream. In reality, I reached eleventh place out of three hundred, and there were only ten places available for non-Italians. My father had died of cancer a year earlier, and there wasn't really anyone or anything to keep me there, so I packed my bags and the remainder of my dignity and returned to Israel to figure out what to do with the rest of my life.

Why am I sharing this story with you? Just to make clear that as of the time of writing these lines, I have a soft spot for doctors. I admire people who choose this profession. To me, practicing medicine is a holy mission, much like social services, special needs education, nursing, and geriatrics. I'm making this point in order to clarify that I have nothing against doctors and that neither the prior chapter dealing with medical indoctrination nor anything else in this book should be construed in this manner.

I have no anger against anyone who takes up the medical profession, including those who treated me. They are over-worked, sacrifice much of their personal and family lives in order to provide the best care they can to their patients within the constraints of the system they operate in, and do all this within a system that does not care about their individual needs and difficulties and is primarily motivated by profits.

A doctor is first of all a human being. As such it is not surprising that the same psychological mechanisms that lead us to anger, irritation, excitement, or repression of emotions, and the same situations that shake people out of their calm or touch something deep in their hearts also apply to physicians.

Doctors also get out on the wrong side of the bed occasionally, fight with their spouses (if they have a chance to see them between shifts), are driven to distraction by their children (again, to the extent they have a chance see them), and get upset with their friends just like the rest of us. They too flagellate themselves for personal and professional failures (only more than we do since for them success and failure often really is a matter of life and death), vent at their bosses behind their backs, and enjoy knocking back a few shots and getting plastered, (hopefully when they aren't on duty), just like you and I do.

Human character comes, of course, in all shapes and sizes. In the case of doctors, their specific character might be expressed in the types of residency they choose. A man who chooses to specialize in geriatrics, and is prepared to help and support individuals in the twilight of their lives and throughout the unique challenges of this period, is essentially different in his outlook and character than an individual who has chosen to mend bones as an orthopedic surgeon.

Both are different from an individual who chooses to specialize in gynecology and insert objects into vaginas all day long, or proctologists who do the same with rear orifices. That gynecologist is quite different in character than the internist who spends his day collecting data about his patients like an intelligence unit analyst, or the surgeon who might be compared to a type of commando operating behind enemy lines. On the other side of this scale are pediatricians, whose decision to assist infants just beginning to make their way through the world is indicative of their gentleness, or oncologists who view their daily struggle against cancer as a type of sacred duty.

To summarize, doctors are human beings, just like you and me. Sometimes they are wrong. Sometimes they make mistakes. And just like you and me, sometimes they don't learn from their mistakes and keep on repeating them until life comes back to bite them and teaches them a thing or two.

Until it does, and until they do, their egos work overtime to prove they were right all along and suppress everything that does not fit the familiar pattern, just like our egos. And, just like you and me, they have better days and worse days and even days where they have no patience for patients and their complaints, and all they want to do is cuddle under their blankets and go back to sleep.

This is the time to put ourselves in the shoes of the average doctor. A powerful inner compulsion to help people get well leads him to spend a huge chunk of his life in medical school and residency, a time that is characterized by days with little or no sleep and blind obedience to senior doctors who don't really think their subordinates have anything new to teach them and are less than enthusiastic to hear anything that deviates from the conventions of the system.

None of this contributes to a doctor's self-confidence as an individual or a medical professional. And then, on top of all that are thousands of shifts in endless loops where he is obliged to toe the policy lines of the medical system. Only once he has completed this path of thorns, and armed with nothing but his mother's satisfaction that her son is finally an accredited doctor (and we certainly should not take that satisfaction lightly), does this typical doctor assume a position in one of the major hospitals, where he finally thinks he has the authority and opportunity to help patients—only to collide face-first into reality.

Before we accompany the doctor in his collision with reality, we must address the issue of emotions in the medical profession, or more accurately the negation of their validity by the system and the profession. While doctors are human beings just like you and me, they have been taught, trained, and conditioned to suppress, ignore, or bury their feelings when they treat patients from the moment they set foot in medical school.

The original reason for this was very practical and sensible—a doctor must know how to control his emotions in order to think, analyze, and operate efficiently under extreme stress conditions when matters of life and death are at stake. There is no disputing this.

In practice, somewhere along this long and rocky road, doctors have become mere mechanics who treat diseases without even seeing their patients as human. This is not merely my opinion; this is the testimony of doctors themselves, or at least those courageous enough to write about it. This relegation to the statues of "disease technicians" leads them slowly but surely to medical fatigue, which is often accompanied by loss of kindness and patience, precisely when their patients most require that kindness, an encouraging word, and above all, hope.

> *We doctors tend to minimize the deeper aspects of the human soul to the point that we treat self-reflection or addressing our own needs as a nearly perverted action… The doctor must overcome his inner resistance, for who can enlighten another when he himself is in darkness? And who can purify another when he himself is not been cleansed?*
>
> —— Karl Jung

And, to illustrate the point, please consider Collision with Reality Exhibit A: An average patient enters the doctor's room in Israel or the UK or almost any other public health medical system that is dedicated to providing medical services to the entire population regardless of socioeconomic differences. He is one of dozens waiting outside, some nervous and impatient because the hospital (or the clinic) allocates five-minute appointments, which is clearly unrealistic, unproductive, and inhumane.

Yet the profit motive as a supreme value overcomes professional and common-sense considerations to the detriment of both physicians and patients. On top of all that, there are always those who never set up an appointment but who just need to "ask one brief question," and they will burst into the doctor's room without asking or being considerate of those who have set up an appointment. (To be sure, the phenomenon of pushing ahead of the queue is perhaps more common in Israel than elsewhere.)

Tucked inside this madhouse is our doctor. A doctor who really does want to help people. A doctor who wants, deep inside, to treat every patient as an individual in order to better understand what they are going through and help them feel better. But he can't. How can he? He is scheduled to see dozens of patients during his shift, the time is pressing, and he needs to carry out a lightning-swift diagnosis during which he needs to take in the patient's account and the various physiological indicators, deal with his various complaints, cross-reference to prior medical information from other specialist practitioners, and carry out a physical examination. Then he needs to process all of this information in order to determine the proper treatment of the medical condition or disease.

Those of my readers who have been spared the above irritations, so typical of tax-funded public health systems, have instead suffered the downsides of the American medical system, in which most healthcare is provided by the private sector, and patients are medically insured through their workplaces or through personal arrangements with private sector insurance companies (at least those fortunate enough to be insured).

The medical bills such individuals receive are much higher and, being the subject of negotiation between their insurance companies and the hospitals (and the hospitals' efforts to include various unnecessary labor and procedures), cannot be calculated in advance. On the other hand, one waits less time to receive medical treatment, and the experience of waiting in line in the hospital is much less chaotic.

Still, as far as the doctor treating you is concerned, it is all the same. He is still under pressure to take in as many patients as possible to maximize the profits of the private companies running the hospital. And as a bonus, he is also under unofficial pressure to administer as many medical procedures as possible. That's how the bills presented to medical insurance, and eventually to the patients, get inflated.

Now imagine in that same time, suddenly the patient lectures **the doctor** about various things he read online and begins pestering him with questions about whether it might be worthwhile to try something else. What would you do at that moment if you were the doctor? Imagine what would go through your head at that point. Most likely it is something like "Just what I need. Another smartass who read something on the internet. Everyone thinks he's a doctor at the click of a mouse."

You would probably dismiss what he had to say, right? Or else you would mutter something like "Do you know the chances of this working? Zero! Do you know how many people try this and fail? Do you even know what this means or what it will require from you?" Or else you might nod and tell him "You are welcome to investigate the matter and get a second opinion. Please call in the next patient on your way out." Not because you have anything against this particular patient, but because you just don't have time for this bullshit right now. Right?

Or imagine that suddenly a patient starts talking about the pressure he has at work or that he has been laid off or how his spouse is always on his case, or that his kids are out of control, or about the grief he feels since his mother passed away. What would go through your head if you were in the doctor's shoes? Something like "Well, why is he burdening me with his problems? I don't have time for this, and it isn't my job to deal with it. Let him go see a shrink. I have thirty other patients outside." This is reality—and it is harsh.

The reality in which physicians work, regardless of the type of medical system they work in (private or public), and the specific country they work in is harsh and characterized by many pressures. Some of them are external. The pharmaceutical companies want to push more and more drugs at the patients, and the hospital administration wants the doctor to perform as many medical procedures as possible, because the insurance companies pay for each procedure separately.

As for the patients, they clamor for this or that drug or medical procedure because they saw it on television or because that is the only way they feel their illness receives a real treatment, regardless of their doctor's professional opinion of the drug or treatment.

Other pressures are internal. Apathy toward the patients, which transforms the doctor into no more than a disease technician, frustrations and anxieties stemming from an inability to help patients (or advance professionally—did I mention that doctors are people too?), and, of course, exhaustion caused by long shifts under time pressure, whether in the clinic or the hospital.

Now let us consider Collision with Reality Exhibit B, in the form of a sympathetic patient hospitalized where our doctor works. A personal connection forms between them. The doctor finds himself listening at length, beyond what is dictated by the standard protocol, to the personal story of the patient and begins to see beyond the numbers, the data, the statistics, and the diagnosis.

This patient and this rare interaction make the doctor try to go the extra mile, beyond what he knows and has been taught, to question and investigate further. They make him—they force him—to feel. But what happens when this enthused doctor approaches his seniors or superiors and shares his feelings, discoveries, findings, and proposals with them? In most cases, he will receive a cold reception in the form of a brutal reminder of his commitment to the protocols of the hospital, to legal liability, and to the procedures and processes of the hospital that are dictated to all new employees of the institute.

Should this doctor continue rocking the boat, this entire arsenal of methods will be used to muzzle him and pull him back into the same narrow furrow that all other hospital employees tread. His head will soon be emptied of "that sort of nonsense." Nothing personal, that's just how the system works. That doctor will soon be back to parroting the medical practitioner cant, the language of diseases that mandates an emotionless and uncaring detachment. Reality is cruel.

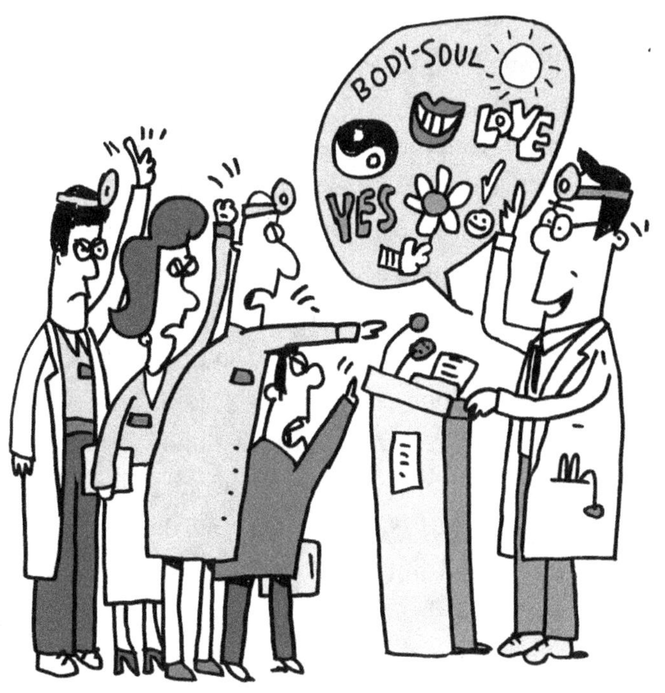

A rebellious doctor studies, investigates, and finds answers that contradict everything his colleagues and coworkers believe in.

Inside the Mind of a Rebellious Doctor

You have probably already wondered "Why is she spending so much time talking about doctors?" and you are right to wonder. Why am I dwelling so much on the subject? Because, paradoxically, it is only thanks to doctors that I was able to successfully cure myself, and only thanks to doctors did I learn that I needed to listen to my own soul if I wanted to cure myself from my own diseases.

But I never met these doctors in the clinics of the mainstream medical system. I never met them in the many hospitals that hosted me over the years. The doctors you meet there are those trained to fight diseases, not help patients get well. I had to actively seek out the second kind of doctors. I had to put a real effort into it and, of course, realize that they existed in the first place.

Before I embarked on this search, I had run into unusual self-curing stories of ex-patients who had succeeded and survived against all odds, and they awakened within me the inspiration and initial will to cure myself and become healthy. Once that desire was kindled within me, the next step—finding these "rebel" doctors—became much easier.

Why do I call them "rebels"? Because each of them turned against the system that made them what they were. The system provided them with their training, education, professional development, and social prestige. More importantly, the system provided them with the terms they used to define themselves. Can you even begin to comprehend how much courage is required to do that? How much mental and spiritual fortitude? The extent of negative reaction received from the environment? The mockery from one's colleagues? And to even get to that point, years of questioning and the self-doubt of asking questions no one around the doctor is prepared to entertain let alone answer must be endured, and the negation of much of the foundation of what the doctor believed in and lived according to must be faced.

And then, after he passes through these stages and finds the answers he was seeking, then realizes that those answers completely contradict everything that he and his colleagues have been taught and all the principles according to which the doctor has lived and worked, the doctor wants to write a book about it and spread the word. After all, the reason he became a doctor in the first place was to help people, and how can the answers he found help people if they remain hidden?

But here's the catch—the rebel's professional future and reputation are at stake. Being a secret heretic is one thing, but the public humiliation and scorn that the scientific community and leading medical institutions will exact upon him are something else entirely. The rebel fears the heavy price he will have to pay for publicly testifying the truth he has found, the truth that is unpalatable to so many people in his professional and social circles. And yet, he still goes public. An internal voice tells him not to let it go, not to give up, to bring the truth into the light.

These brave rebel doctors come from all fields of modern medicine, from genetics to psychiatry, and from all parts of the world. Thanks to them, I have successfully completed my long journey toward pill-free health, and it is thanks to their myriad journeys that I have been able to write this book. Some of the materials appearing in this volume are summaries or direct quotations from the books they wrote, the lectures they delivered, or the documentaries in which they appear.

It is they who are the wise men of science. I am no doctor, but by listening to them, I gained the validation and faith that I could try and succeed, and I eventually did. You can, too. They are out there. Look for them. Be active and take responsibility. It is a central part of your own healing process.

The way forward is simple, but it is far from easy. We may not be doctors, and will therefore not be the primary target of mockery by the medical community, but others certainly will turn their scorn upon us. Many will try to turn us from the path of self-healing, whether driven by their own fears or out of genuine or feigned concern for us. Some will make us feel that we have gone mad, that we are off our rockers, especially when the going gets tough and painful. And, as I mentioned, you will suffer pain and doubt along the way. But if you have faith, you can succeed.

Are you ready to rebel against your disease? Do you understand that the disease is no more than a physiological expression of an internal burden, be it an unresolved pain from the past or a still-active conflict?

PART 2

THE GUIDE TO SELF-HEALING

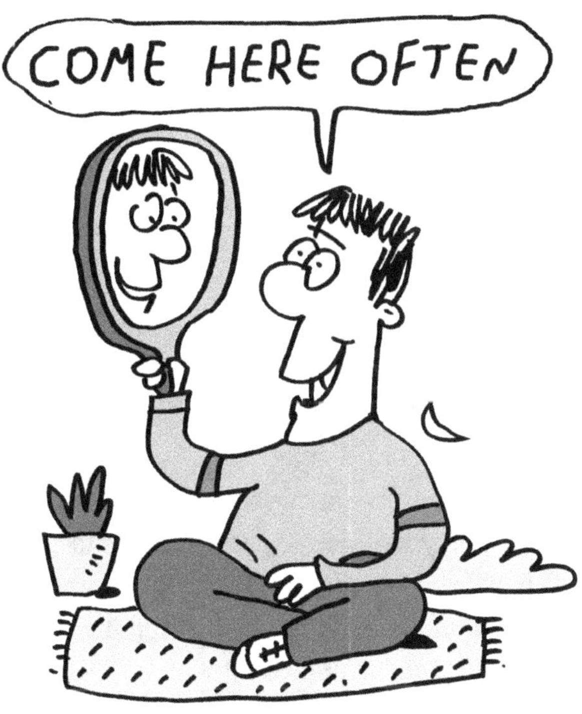

Self-love is the key to all problems in life, small and large. You must learn to truly love yourself.

EIGHT KEYS TO SELF-HEALING (WITH A SPOILER)

Congratulations! you have reached the guide to self healing. If you have done this, something within you must truly want to get well, really wants to get rid of the pills, and is truly open to listen to new things, even if they touch a raw nerve or are challenging, possibly resulting in anger or testiness.

This is where you get the straight dope, or at least the keys to it, since no one can really tell you what your path is or how you personally can reach a life without pills—not me or anyone else on the planet. Why? Because that is how the system works on our planet. No, I didn't invent the rules, so there is no point in complaining to me. Not that I mind if you do—go ahead, blame me for all your many troubles! But that won't really help you in advancing toward your goal; all it will do is make you feel momentarily better about yourself. If you reached this point in the book, I think you probably want more than that. I'm not wrong, am I?

So who can tell you the way to self-healing? Only you. You will have to find it on your own through investigation, questioning, and trial and error. The eight keys that will be detailed in the next chapters will organize your mind about what you need to do and what channels you can work in, will outline a framework to operate in, will guide you on your way, and will give you strength to continue when you run into obstacles and are on the verge of despair. They will empower you to a level you cannot even imagine at the moment, if you choose to act according to them and believe in them.

What they won't do, however, is tell you the specific path that will lead you to health. They will give you macro tools to help you identify and walk the path, but not the micro tools for application in the field—those you will have to work out on your own.

One small bit of encouragement—you won't really be on your own, because if you apply these keys to your life, you will find the sources (human and non-human) that will support you and ensure you never feel alone on the way. Just as important, you will find a part of yourself that has been dormant for many years, even decades—a part of you that you have had no communication with because you have never heard about it, because you have forgotten about it, or because you have suppressed its existence.

That part has repeatedly tried, with little success, to make contact with you, but your sensors didn't register it and you couldn't hear it. Since you couldn't hear, you did not listen, and it had no choice but to utilize harsher means to *make* you listen. Those harsh means were the illnesses you are suffering from, because that was the only way of communication it could employ to get your attention. It moved from whispering to screaming.

You probably guessed that this part is your soul. Once you make a decision to relate to it, when you listen to it and what it has to tell you and when you accept it as part of you, that is when you will be able to feel whole again. At that point, you will no longer feel alone, because you will have all of yourself. And that, friends, is a gift just as valuable as your physical health, as I can personally attest to.

WATCH OUT, SPOILER AHEAD

Here comes the spoiler I promised. Do you know what will happen after you undergo this process and learn to connect with and bond with this part within you? The most worn-out cliché is what will happen—you will be able to begin to love yourself again. I am not talking about love that is all in your mind, my friends, or telling the whole world how much you love yourself, shopping yourself to death, living the good life, and then harming yourself quietly when you are alone with food that is bad for you, gambling, addictions, bad couple relations, drugs (legal or illegal), self-cutting, not listening to yourself, or any of the other thousands of creative ways people can use to inflict harm on themselves when they are bound and determined to do so.

What I am talking about here is love that you can feel in your heart. You will be in a place where you say, "I love myself. I am crazy about myself," and it will be the truth, not an empty mantra to repeat to yourself. Not a mask for the outside world.

How will you know this is the truth? Because the love

will be expressed in hundreds of everyday actions, and not just in talk. You really will be able to look at yourself in the mirror, even in the nude—with your belly fatand your sagging post-nursing breasts—and feel that you really love yourself as you are.

So why do I consider this cliché to be a spoiler? Because self-love is the key to all problems in life, large or small. I am sorry, my friends, that I have no novel news, but just the same old cliché that we have all heard thousands of times in twenty-one thousand different pop songs. (Who sang "All you need is love" and didn't get it?) Terribly disappointing, isn't it? What a bummer, right? Why can't there be some innovative magic solution that none of us has ever heard of that can be bought (preferably online without breaking a sweat), then swallowed and leads us to wake up to a better world where we are all healthy and happy?

With the same certainty, I am telling you that self-love is the key to all of our problems in life. I am telling you that at least 95 percent of the people in Western society don't really love themselves, and it has nothing to do with how much money they have, how advanced and successful they are at their jobs, how tall, skinny, and pretty they are, or what they tell their circles of friends and family. And no, it doesn't really matter what country or city they live in. The grass isn't greener on the other side.

If you could sit with any one of them and have a true and honest discussion, you would find out that none of them really love themselves, that each of them has problems with themselves, that they all have inner conflicts, bad habits, and parts that they would love to change or exchange with someone else.

How can I be so sure of something that was never conclusively, scientifically proven? Because over the past decade, I have studied the subject in depth, since I had dozens of questions I wanted answered. I have studied the words of wise men and spiritual leaders who lived on this planet centuries and millennia ago, all over the world, in eras when there was no internet or any significant intercontinental communication, and they still talked about the same things.

True, they used different words in different languages and with different associations, colors, and metaphors (after all their cultures were very different). But essentially, they were all speaking of the same issues. That these words of wisdom were retained to this day and are accessible to anyone who is prepared to peruse them is an indication of the timelessness of their messages.

Besides listening to wise people from the past, and quite a few wise people from the present, who help millions of people all over the world, I have read about, listened to, and watched dozens of doctors and scientists with conventional training, from all fields and sub-fields of life sciences and from countries all over the world, who have reached the same conclusion in one way or another. I have personally interviewed dozens of people who escaped the grip of the angel of death in spite of conventional medicine condemning them to die, and have read of thousands of others from all over the world of all races, genders, and religions.

The millions of words that I have read and the thousands

of hours I have spent watching lectures and documentaries of scientists and other wise people have lesser weight on my convictions than what I discovered by myself, on myself. I was both the scientist and the guinea pig, the lab rat with all the knowledge I acquired over an extremely long process of study, experimentation, and error. that I applied, until I was finally successful in healing myself and living a healthy and balanced life without the aid of chemical pills.

If I had to answer with a short sentence the question "What did you learn during all these years?," then the answer is that I learned to love myself. Self-love is the key to healing, the key to happiness, the key to acceptance, the key to inner peace, and the key to connecting ourselves to who we essentially are on the deepest level.

It was scientifically proven a long time ago that even our genes respond to love on the physiological-biochemical-cellular level. It has also been scientifically proven that our genes respond negatively, insofar as the effects on our physiology are concerned, to hatred and its various expressions. (Dr. Bruce Lipton details in his book, *The Biology of Belief* a wide variety of such studies.)

Experiments by Masaru Emoto have even showed that thoughts, words, and ideas affect the molecular structure of water. When you consider that over 70 percent of our bodies are made up of water, you can well imagine the physical effect of words upon us. It has been proven that self-hatred weakens the body's immune system.

And what happens when the system that safeguards us from invasion weakens? That's right, we get sick and infected with pathogens. Ever wonder why two people can be exposed to the same infection in the same room, but one leaves healthy and the other is infected by a virus and bedridden for several days? What happens when the weakened immune system persists for many years? That's right, that's how chronic diseases develop.

Testing, Testing

Here are two small, simple exercises that can help you begin to find out just how much self-love you have. I must note that although these exercises are very simple to understand, they are not particularly easy to apply and some of you might find it very hard or nearly impossible to perform. Perhaps that difficulty might be good in and of itself, since this could be a first step toward understanding that there might be a few things you should do to feel better about yourself. That understanding might, in turn, lead you step-by-step to a healthier life. There will be many steps along the way, but the first step is sometimes the hardest and most important.

The first exercise is a classic mirror exercise.[1] Stand in front of the mirror for thirty days, every day. The time of day or type of mirror you stand in front of don't matter— the important thing is to do this when you are alone. Look straight into your reflection's eyes and declare confidently, "I

---

1   I first learned about the mirror exercise from the excellent book by Louise Hay, *You Can Heal Your Life*.

love you." Say this thirty times each day.

That is the seemingly easy part of the exercise. **The more challenging part is to be conscious of what occurs on the physical, emotional, or behavioral levels when you do this.** Can you successfully perform the exercise? Do you get stuck after a few repetitions? Do you find it easy or difficult? Can you feel the love in your heart or can't you? What feelings rise up in you when you say "I love you" to yourself? Good feelings like happiness, excitement, wonderment, and acceptance? Or less pleasant emotions like anger, disappointment, fear, sadness, impatience, lack of clarity, fear, vulnerability, and loneliness? What kinds of thoughts do you have when you say "I love you"? Positive thoughts like "What fun!" or "I am lucky!" or less sympathetic thoughts such as "This is stupid," "You're lying," "I don't believe you," "You are unworthy of love," or even "You idiot"?

The second exercise is also thirty days long, and it is performed by asking a very simple question about situations, interpersonal encounters, or challenging moments in our everyday lives.

In every situation where you find yourself debating what to do, what to say, how to behave, what to choose, or how to respond, ask yourself the following question: "What would a person who loves himself do?"[2]

Our lives are filled with hundreds of everyday situations, some of them repetitive, where we interact with people

---

2   I learned about this charming exercise at a lecture by the spiritual teacher Teal Swan.

and need to respond in a certain way because that is what is expected of us, because that is our job, or because that is just how life is. For example, your boss might blame you for something you didn't do, or yell at you or berate you in front of a colleague. A good friend might be disappointed because you don't call him often enough. A parent might use emotional blackmail to get you to do something while ignoring your desires. A significant other might treat you disrespectfully, whether by word or by deed (up to and including emotional and physical abuse).

An opportunity arises to travel to an event with long-unmet friends, but your child is sick and your husband is sour about it. A desire to learn something new or sign up for a certain class. Endless situations with children that challenge us to provide nonstop giving, while forgetting that it is both possible and desirable to get something back. (And I'm not talking about wanting to sleep throughout the night while the child wakes up ten times during the night.)

Whenever you encounter one of these situations, ask yourself this: "What would a person who truly loved himself do?" Ask yourself this once a day, twice, five times, or even ten times a day and see what comes up. Where is there resistance? What are the thoughts popping up automatically? How do I feel about them? Does the answer to this question make me change my reaction in practice? Did I suddenly behave differently because I asked the question?

After thirty days, we can get a pretty good idea of how attentive we are to ourselves and respond or act from that place. We get an idea of how aware we are of our needs and desires, and to what extent we allow ourselves to respond to and realize them. At the end of the day, a significant part of self-love is attentiveness to the self, to our true needs and desires whenever and wherever one can.

So whether you choose to perform these nice exercises or not, my declaration stands: **The gateway to healing and a healthy, pill-free life is self-love.** Sorry, friends, there is no escaping it. If you want to be healthy, you will have to learn to love yourself with a true love. **The way to health goes through the heart. There are no shortcuts or bypasses.**

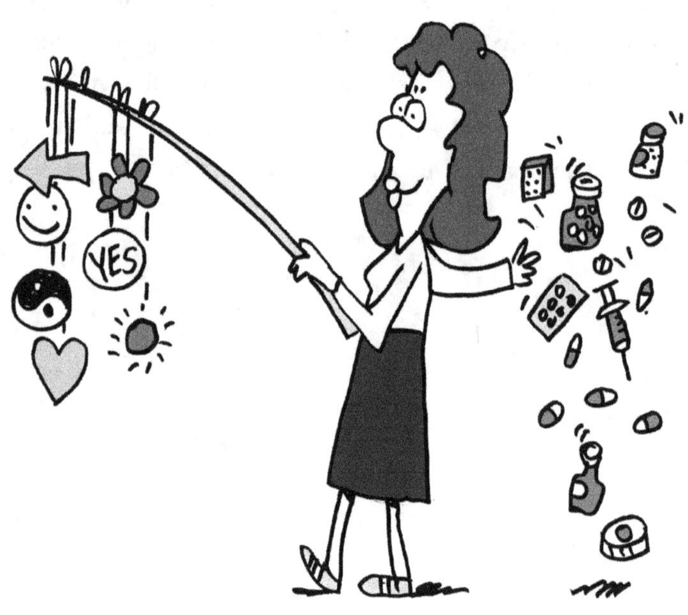

Faith is the first gateway you must pass. You must truly believe yourself in order to be capable of healing yourself.

WE CAN CURE OURSELVES FROM DISEASE

"To know the path before you, ask the people who have walked it."

— Chinese proverb

It all begins and ends with faith. Faith is the first gateway that you must pass. You must truly believe yourself to be capable of healing yourself. If you don't believe, there is no point in embarking on the journey. May as well save yourself the disappointment and the distress. Best to stay on the pills instead. That's fine. "To every thing there is a season, and a time to every purpose," as the Old Testament says.

How can this faith be germinated, grown, or developed? There are two places where you can start: the first is the success stories of others, and the second is a deep investigation of the placebo effect.

Before I detail these two planes, this is the place to remind you once again of the three indoctrinations we who live in Western society are subject to.

1. Modern medicine is all about curing diseases.
2. Doctors know all there is to know about how to cure all diseases, chronic diseases included.
3. Diseases are genetic.

You are invited to reread chapter 2, where this indoctrination is detailed, since these three insidious memes will constantly pop up and disrupt the self-healing process, so deeply have they been embedded into our psyches. We have learned to accept them as facts, to breathe with them, to live with them, to look at the world through them, to analyze with them.

Questioning this indoctrination will sometimes feel like we are fighting ourselves, which is odd and will even lead us to question ourselves. "How is it that connection to myself is accompanied by such a strong sense of separation?" The answer is that saying goodbye to old beliefs may be deeply rewarding, but it is also super-challenging. The only effective way to deal with these sensations is to constantly remind ourselves that it is possible to deal with them, via two tactics on which I will now expand.

The success stories of others are an excellent starting point. Reading about the journeys of other people who have succeeded against all odds, and against everything their doctors told them, to cure themselves can lift your spirits. It doesn't matter what chronic or terminal diseases they cured themselves of. **That is where you will find the will to make it happen, the faith that it is possible, the courage to try, and the ability to set your feet upon the path.** The feeling that you are not alone in this story (even though most of the time you will be alone on the journey of self-healing).

You will know that others walked this path before you, that others dared to hope and pray. That others overcame every obstacle and barrier. This feeling is invaluable, and can be a matter of life and death for those whom the conventional medical system had given up on and condemned to death. They can testify to this, for many of them are still with us, years after their death sentence.

Hearing these people speak and share the hardships of their journeys—what helped them, what kept their spirits up, what brought them low, and what helped them get back on their feet after every time that they stumbled on the way, how they felt to get their lives back, and how it feels to love and appreciate themselves for the long road they traveled—hearing all this will touch you deep inside, and the effect will only grow, the more success stories you read or hear about.

You may even meet people who have walked the path of self-healing and hear them share their experience face-to-face, helping you build up your faith in your ability to walk in their footsteps. You will come to feel that you, just as much as they, deserve to be and are capable of being healthy. You do deserve to live a life without pills. That is the path to walk.

That's Them, not Me

If, on the other hand, you find that these tales of success depress rather than uplift you, and make you feel bad about yourself because "others are better than I am, and I'm just not good enough to succeed" or "Just because they made it doesn't mean I can" or "Nothing I ever do works," then it is better that you don't try right now. Better to let go for now. Until you feel a burning desire to succeed within you, there is no point to embarking on the path to self-healing.

It's a hard enough road as it is, filled with challenges, disappointments, repeated attempts, and frustrations. Not everyone can take them in stride. Even with faith and flaming desire, handling those obstacles and reversals is hard. The path is long and torturous.

Don't feel bad about it. Don't feel there is something wrong with you. Five years went by between the moment the thought occurred to me that I wanted to live without pills to the moment I decided to embark on the path to make that desire reality. And each one of those years was necessary to prepare me for the journey.

You should keep reading about the healing journeys of others, but do so from the perspective of being on a research tour of the possibility of opening up to the maybe. "Maybe I can do this. Maybe I can take action and realize my desires."

Right now, you're just studying the subject in detail. If you are ill with a chronic autoimmune disease and are taking pills, there is no pressure at all, so take your time. If the angel of death is banging on your door, that is a different story entirely, but also one that gives you something of an advantage—you really don't have a choice.

If you truly love life, or have rediscovered your love of life thanks to the disease and understand that you are not prepared to give up, if you really want to be healthy (and not just to stop being sick, two entirely different things), then good morning and Godspeed! Have faith in yourself and be on your way.

Many people will tell you that the success stories of others are no indication of your statistical chances of success and they, of course, will be right. Many doctors will tell you that these success stories are a minority and that most people fail and die. (Or in the case of chronic diseases, just stay on the pills until they die. Ironic, don't you think?) And yes, they too are right.

So the questions arise: **Which story do you choose to live? Who do you choose to be? Do you choose to be the minority who succeeds and lives? Do you choose to be a success story? Deep inside, do you believe that you, like all the others who succeeded, can make it as well? If the answer is positive, you are cordially invited to take responsibility for yourself and your disease and set off on your path to self-healing.**

I want to make one final point to sum up this part. The phrase "we can cure ourselves of diseases" is not scientifically proven. There is no actual scientific proof that people can cure themselves from diseases. And I have news for you: It will never be scientifically proven. Why? Because there is no one to research the issue and prove it. Why? Because there is no money in it.

Over the years, leading scientific and medical journals have published thousands of case studies of people being cured from a vast variety of diseases, but they have all been titled with the sexy moniker of "spontaneous recoveries."

This title means that yes, there is acknowledgement of a remarkable recovery taking place, but it has no explanation other than being a remarkable story.

You might ask, "Why has no one risen to the challenge and investigated the matter more deeply if these stories repeat themselves in various permutations?" That's right, the answer is that those who have the massive funds and resources to support such scientific studies are not interested in doing so. What would they patent? What would they register as an exclusive intellectual right? Proper nutrition? Mental health? Spiritual growth? Love of self? Attentiveness to the voice of the soul?

You can't make money out of any of those things, and so no money is invested in researching them. That is how the medical system is rigged in Western society. The industry only makes money if we are ill. If we are healthy, they lose money. Do you know a single corporation that is in the business of losing money? There is no such beast.

So even though the axiom of "we can heal ourselves" has not and will not be scientifically proven, each and every one of you can read these stories and reach your own decision about whether they inspire you to action or whether it seems nonsense or the luck that only other people have.

PRIMORDIAL SELF-HEALING ABILITIES

There is, as I earlier mentioned, a second source of inspiration and faith in your ability to heal yourself, and it *is* scientifically proven. This is the placebo effect. Personally, I believe that the placebo is a gift we receive from our creator, meant to demonstrate to us how the body is capable of curing itself from any situation, pain, or disease. It shows how this primordial self-healing ability is imprinted in our body's very essence, regardless of whether we believe in it, dismiss it, use it, or prove it scientifically.

A placebo effect occurs on two levels. The first is when a patient receives a treatment with no active ingredient (like a sugar pill or a water injection), and his condition still improves. In other words, the effect is actually one of a dummy cure on a patient who believes he received "real" medicine.

The second level on which the placebo effect operates is expectation. You achieve this by exposing people to a sort of suggestion, such as "From now on, you will not feel any pain" or "Your blood pressure will improve." The expectation shifts their brain chemistry. For this reason, many doctors prescribe placebos to anxious patients in the hope that this will relieve their anxieties. In other words, the beliefs of an individual about the healing powers of the treatment catalyze the activation of physiological systems to promote recovery.

So what is this all about? A man believes that he will recover thanks to a medical intervention and yes, he recovers…but no actual medical intervention took place! The body arranged the matters on its own and functioned as an independent pharmacy without any actual chemical intervention by exterior forces. If it looks like a duck, walks like a duck, and quacks like a duck, then it's as good as a duck—or better.

The placebo effect scientifically proves that faith can have just as much effect as the active ingredient in medication, that the mind can overcome the matter, and that each of us has an inbuilt pharmacy. The percent of "magic" performed by the placebo effect is 30 percent, not 100 percent, so the body cures itself on its own only in a third of the cases when the "dummy" medicine is not accompanied by "real" medicine. But some studies have shown improvement, if not full recovery, in 100 percent of the cases.

It is recommended that you study the field and be inspired by it. Let your body inspire you. Given the proper conditions, it will know how to cure itself. In other words, you will be able to cure yourself if you only believe in its abilities.

This leads me to my summary of the first key to self-healing: If—after you understand that you have been indoctrinated in regard to everything relating to the world of modern medicine, read the success stories of others, and dig into the wonders of the placebo effect—you hear an inner voice telling you that yes, you can, then listen to it. Listen to yourself. Believe in yourself, believe in your body and its inbuilt powerful ability, and provide it with the ideal conditions to prove it to you. Most people will silence this voice very quickly, and that's fine—for them. The question is, which group of people do you belong to?

Summary of the First Key

- Remember that we are all indoctrinated in regard to Western medicine.
- You must believe that you can cure yourself from diseases.
- Read about the various success stories.
- Study and learn about the placebo effect.

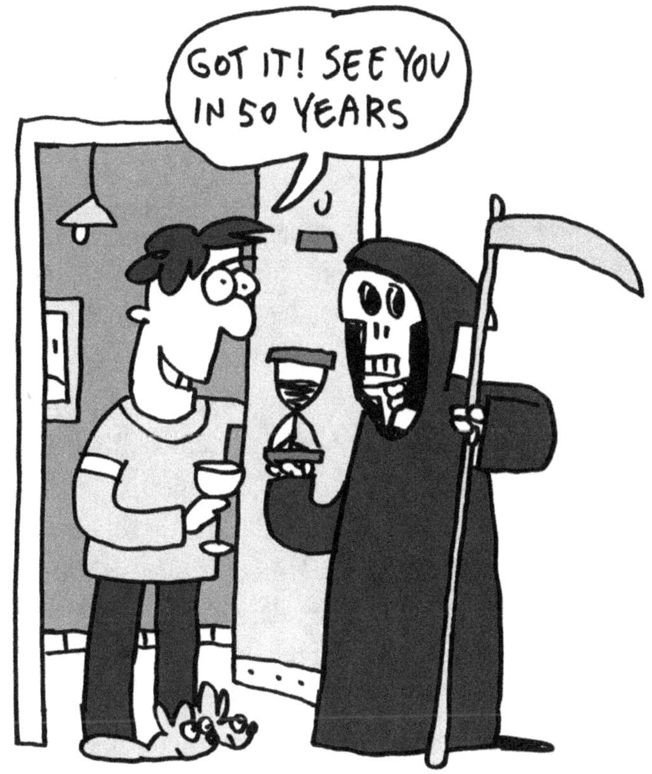

Disease is an opportunity to transition from "Oh, no. This is terrible," to "Oh my God! What an opportunity!"

DISEASE IS A TOOL OF HEALING

Friends, we are all screwed up in one way or another. If there is a screw-up scale between one and ten, 99.99 percent of humanity is on it somewhere. In our imbalanced and stressful Western society, most of us are on the upper rungs of that scale, both mentally injured and physically ill. We are all carrying the baggage of internal traumas; that is how it works here on Earth, and no one is exempt.

All of us have to deal with the deaths of loved ones (family or friends); breakups (whether by our initiative or not, justified or not, easy or hard); failures (in our careers, academic studies, or personal lives); abandonment (by our parents, significant others, or our children); sexual abuse (in childhood or adulthood); or even physical harm (incapacity, diseases, or accidents).

Every one of these traumas leaves its emotional-mental imprint upon us, and many of them scar us for life. To keep things interesting, the long-term scars are overshadowed by everyday anxieties, which accompany us every day and every hour, like bosom buddies looking out for us.

When you get right down to it, it is not easy being a human. From the very first second that we are separated from the warm and comforting space of our mother's womb and are exposed to the blinding fluorescent lighting of the delivery room, we must face down one emotionally tumultuous encounter after another, and it only gets worse as time goes by.

Some of these encounters hurt. Hurt badly. Not on the physical level of "I fell down, scraped my knee. Ouch, I hurt. Mommy, give me a kiss to make it better." No, it agonizes our very soul. We generally don't get what we want because what we want is not healthy, not appropriate, not fair, not cheap, not possible, or not available. What we do get is many ringing slaps to our face.

You don't have to grow up in an orphanage or find out that you are adopted in order to feel abandoned and neglected. A child can feel that way when he grows up with parents who work for many hours outside the house, or with parents who are present but are busy on the phone or with other things.

You don't need to have abusive parents who put out cigarettes on your skin, beat you, or sexually molest you to be emotionally scarred. A child can feel that way even when a "more successful" sibling is treated better, or when he is told repeatedly that he is a liar or a wimp who will "never amount to anything," who "no one will want to be with," who is "no good at anything," or who "thinks too highly" of himself.

He can be emotionally scarred by not being sufficiently hugged or given loving physical contact. These harsh feelings also arise when you grow up in a normal or seemingly normal house, and they hurt us. Badly. We don't want to feel this pain, so we suppress it, along with the reasons for it.

EMOTIONAL MEMORIES

Suppression is a type of survival mechanism that helps us move on with our life in spite of the pain and emotional injury. This mechanism serves us well and works splendidly, with the exception of one small problem—our conscious mind may forget or deny and move on, surviving the trauma and going on with its life as if nothing had occurred.

But "as if" are the key words here. In reality, the trauma did occur and did hurt, humiliate, and tear you up inside. The conscious mind might forget, but the soul never forgets what happened and the body never forgets what happened, and they cannot be fooled. These painful memories are preserved in every cell of our bodies. They are called emotional memories, and they run our life through our automatic reactions to people, places, and situations.

Many of us have had the experience of passing by a place where something unpleasant happened to us in the past, even if many years have passed since the event, and immediately experiencing physiological responses such as cramps, rapid breathing, increased heartbeat, or shivering, as if it had happened yesterday. Many of us have also responded to the voice of a person who has offended us in the past, by putting our body into a defensive stance.

Even certain smells can trigger similar responses. For example, if something unpleasant had happened to me in a place with a powerful odor of tulips, it is quite likely that I would have a hard time enjoying the smell of tulips in the future. If someone who used a given perfume offended me, whether once or systematically over a long period of time, chances are that when I run into that particular perfume again, those same harsh sensations they made me feel will rise within me again. The body remembers both the physical burdens (and their actual means of expression) and the mental burdens (the entire range of emotions and thoughts we felt during that traumatic event).

Do you ever find yourself behaving differently than what you intend or are accustomed to in non-traumatic situations, speaking differently than what you would want or are used to, or responding differently than you want or are accustomed to? For example, have you found yourself exploding at someone on account of silly nonsense with zero significance? If you have, then odds are that there is something buried deep within that is painful and unresolved that has nothing to do with that person or situation, or is related to your history with the person you exploded at but not the specific situation you are exploding at.

In short, you have made a fool of yourself without really understanding how or why, and are unable to control yourself. It is very easy to identify this in arguments or fights between couples. When a couple is fighting over who will clear out the garbage, they aren't really fighting over removing the stinking garbage bag. When a couple is fighting over the excessive expenses of one member or whether the toilet seat is up or down or the lousy performance of their children in school, what they are really fighting about is much deeper than that specific issue.

Aspects of fear, anger, miscommunication, attentiveness, feeling insulted, hatred, low self-esteem, and other such nuggets are all there. Each of us has our own personal scars in our personal biographies. They follow us everywhere, 24/7 (yes, even in our dreams), and they run our lives.

Mind and Body Are Truly One

Once we have realized how the body and the soul remember, even when the conscious mind forgets, it is time to move on to the next stage. Who among us cannot recite that "mind and soul are one," or as men wiser than I have said, "A healthy mind is a healthy body"?

We all know that if our body is feeling poorly, our soul aches as well, because when we are ill, we feel bad. We even know that if we feel bad emotionally, the body will respond accordingly in the form of illness or fatigue. But what do we actually do the second something hurts? We forget about all that knowledge and run off to get some medication to ease our pain. "Doctor, doctor! Help me, I'm hurting!" The pain upsets our judgment, and we will do anything to relieve it, make it disappear, and never come back.

Now, I'm not saying you should be masochistic and cling to the pain. Not at all. I'm just trying to turn your attention toward the fact that when we run off to take a pill that will relieve the pain, we are making life easy for ourselves in the short run but harming ourselves in the long run, since we are ignoring the natural mechanism, which we all can recite like parrots, but which we fail to implement at the moment of truth.

The mechanism is simple. It tells us that when the body is in pain, the soul is in pain, and when the body is ill, the soul is ill. The body and soul are dependent on each other and maintain, just like two organisms in nature, a symbiotic relationship where there is close attachment, partnership, and codependence.

So before you take the pill, ask yourself, "What is this pain here to tell me? What is my soul trying to tell me?" Once you swallow that pill, the pain will be gone, but so will the message of the soul and desire to find out the deeper cause for the pain.

That is how we are—we forget quickly, but when we start hurting, we cannot forget that our soul is the source and reason for the pain. That is the practical meaning of this key, and it requires a certain amount of self-awareness. We won't always get immediate online answers to our queries. You shouldn't expect to release a question to the air about the source of the pain and immediately come up with an answer.

It might happen that simply raising the issue into our

consciousness will reveal the solution, but sometimes the answer is not apparent on the surface and needs to be sought after. You must be patient during the discovery process, and consciously follow the developments and the circumstances of your illness. Neutralizing the cause will neutralize the painful outcome.

We proceed stage by stage, and the stage following the pain is the disease. **A disease is a physiological symptom of the language of the soul, a chronology of ongoing and system-wide imbalance.** A disease appears after a period in which we have ignored preliminary signs (physiological signs such as pain, changes to our blood pressure, cramps, or rashes, and mental signs such as dreams or nightmares) or alternately that the time has come to emotionally confront the painful sources of the disease.

Diseases develop and evolve over time. Nothing comes from nothing, and nothing appears overnight. There is no hocus pocus in a disease. Our soul has been calling to us, but we have sealed our ears; it has signaled to us and been ignored. It has shouted at us with a megaphone. And when it resorted to pain? We took our pills. Who did this? Our body and our soul, with the soul calling the shots and the body implementing them.

WHAT AN OPPORTUNITY!

Now we come to the real fun, the reason we have gathered here together over the pages of this book. Are you ready?

Here we go.

Disease is a chance to wake up and mobilize ourselves. This is the point in our lives where we can push the envelope (even if for some of us it is a crazy quantum leap), from "Oh no, oh no, woe onto me" to "Wow! This is an incredible opportunity that the disease has given me!"

I am aware that this sounds horrible, especially when you first hear it or if you found out that you or your loved ones suffer from a serious, even terminal, illness. But if you truly wish to increase your chances of recovery, full health, and living out the rest of your life to its fullest, it doesn't really matter which type of treatment you have selected— conventional, alternative, or integrated. To make it work, you absolutely must wake up.

Wake up from what, you ask? From the coma you have been living in without even being aware of it. Why weren't you aware of it? Because not only were you not taught about it, but what you were taught was that diseases are solved by swallowing a pill. Nothing could be further from the truth.

When patients who were ill with cancer were examined, it was found that all of them, without exception, had unresolved inner conflicts. All of them had experienced traumas at some stage or another in their lives that had been treated improperly, or not at all. In other words, their problems were shoved down to the depths of their subconscious. The heavy and dusty dungeon doors were slammed and locked shut, and the torches leading the way were snuffed out.

This is what doctors who have dedicated their lives to treating cancer patients, and who have seen this pattern repeat itself in patient after patient, say. They have never seen a patient who fully accepted himself, who was connected and attentive to himself and his true desires, or who had no untreated past traumas.

I want to stress yet again that **traumas are not exclusive to childhood.** An ugly divorce or breakup is a trauma, as is the death of a parent or a good friend. A prolonged period of stress is also traumatic to the body and the soul. Each and every one of us is unique and each of us responds differently to difficult circumstances on the emotional, mental, physical, and spiritual levels.

Andreas Moritz, who treated thousands of patients and accompanied quite a few cancer patients, defined cancer as "the last attempt of the body to return to life." I invite you to halt for a moment, read that sentence again, and let it echo. Do you realize the depth of this sentence? How much pain it contains, yet at the same time, how much hope and optimism?

WHEN NO CHOICE REMAINS

Do you find this phrase too hard? I invite you to return to my recommendation from the first key and listen to patients who overcame their illnesses. Hear how each of them defines their disease; they define it as the best thing that ever happened to them. Dealing with the disease awakened them and led them to self-attentiveness, to clarify their true desires and to realize them. This led them to self-love, and mostly reminded them how precious and important life is, in all of its myriad layers.

It is actually easier for terminal patients to hear this challenging sentence. It may be the exact opposite of what we would think, but at the end of the day, they have no choice. The angel of death had knocked on their door. "Knock, knock, I'm here. Get ready, say your goodbyes, pack your bags, and move along to a world that is all good."

So some of the people listen to him, because it is frightening, it is threatening, it is paralyzing. Because it might be time to go, because it is better to make use of the time left to say goodbye to loved ones, to make peace with a brother one had not spoken to in over a decade, and perhaps even to perform a bungee jump.

But other people, a second after the stinging slap, zero in on themselves and tell the angel of death, "You think you are taking me? You think I'm coming with you? You must not realize who you are dealing with. Get out of here and don't come back for at least forty years." And then they start the fight of their lives, with all means fair and foul. They miss no chance—all channels of treatment are relevant for them, all options are open, no treatment (no matter how odd) too distasteful. They leave no stone unturned. But what they mostly do is take responsibility for their disease and their life. They choose life.

The medical establishment had given up on them on the therapeutic level and they choose to give it the finger. "What do you mean I'm going to die in a month or two? I don't want to die. What are you going to do, make me?"

These powerful and brave people, who survive against all odds, eventually thank the angel of death for his visit. They thank him for waking them up from the coma, and some of them even write books about the journey they went through, in order to help other people on their own paths and provide them with courage and hope.

All of the above is not exclusive to cancer patients. Cancer is simply one of the most frightening diseases of the twenty-first century because we perceive it as near-certain death. This is also true for patients ill with other chronic diseases. Just because few people in the Western world die immediately from most chronic diseases doesn't mean they do not pose an incredible opportunity for self-healing.

It is true that embarking on the path is harder when no threat of imminent death is hanging over your head, but if we are prepared to listen to our souls speaking to us through chronic illnesses, understand their roles, and be brave enough to face the stories and secrets they drag out of the forgotten dungeons of our souls, chronic diseases can still provide wonderful tools to cure our minds and souls.

SUMMARY OF THE SECOND KEY

- Even if our conscious mind has forgotten or suppressed knowledge in order to protect us from pain, the mind and body remember.
- When the body starts feeling pain, you must not forget that the source and reason for the pain is your soul.
- Diseases develop and incubate over time.

- Use the disease to develop greater attentiveness to your soul, to define your true desires, to realize them, and to remind yourself how precious and important life is.

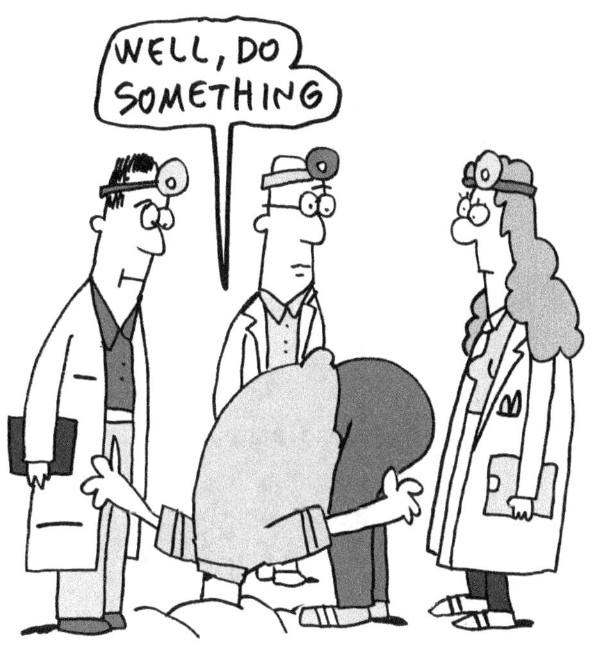

Blaming others makes us focus on other people, and when we commit to self-healing we need to focus on ourselves.

ASSUMING PERSONAL RESPONSIBILITY FOR YOUR DISEASE

Whoever wants to heal himself, recover from illness he has created, and live a healthy life without pills, injections, or various prescription and nonprescription drugs must assume responsibility for doing so. This responsibility is divided into two parts: responsibility for creating the disease in the first place and responsibility for curing it. Both parts are equal in importance and neither can be neglected or overemphasized at the expense of the other.

In the previous chapter, you reviewed how our conscious minds, in order to protect and relieve us from burdens we cannot handle, forget all the bad or unpleasant things that happened to us and hurt us, unlike our bodies and souls, which forget nothing. You also reviewed what we all know but have a hard time implementing in the moment of truth, that our bodies and minds are one and their means of expression are cooperative. Finally, you understood that the creation of a disease is an ongoing process and that a disease is actually a physiological expression of the language of the soul.

It is therefore easier now to reach the derived conclusion: **We are the creators of our own diseases. Or rather a part of us that is usually injured and in pain created the disease, and therefore if we want to cure ourselves, we must take responsibility for it. Responsibility for our own creation.**

It is important to emphasize that taking responsibility is not the same as self-blame, and there is neither cause for nor benefit from self-flagellation. **The processes that create diseases are subconscious.** The entire process occurs without any awareness on our part, just as we are not aware of the various autonomous systems in our bodies that operate 24/7, minute by minute, second by second, with us or without us.

So there is no reason to berate ourselves for making ourselves ill. That doesn't mean you can't do it if you really feel like it, but it would be rather pointless. We blame ourselves for quite enough nonsense as it is, to no benefit in any event, and this just separates us from ourselves even more and leads us to hate ourselves. Paradoxically, and rather sadly, this is one of the most basic and deepest issue that the overall message the soul sends to us through our disease is concerned with. We must learn to love ourselves as we are, with all our supposed flaws, vulnerabilities, anger, fear, and insults from others.

It is sometimes very hard, but it is not impossible. If you are slightly depressed from all this, this is the time to illuminate the positive side of the story. **Just as you created the disease, even if by a subconscious process, so too can you create health.** If there is a reason for this disease and its source can be touched, it is likewise possible to release it from its role and say farewell to it. If the disease is here to tell a story (the story of my soul), and I choose to listen to the story (listen to my soul), I have already done the lion's share of the healing process.

For some patients, that is sufficient. For others, it is not, and they will have to operate in additional channels to achieve health. But to do so, they must assume responsibility for the creation of the disease and for the restoration of balance to their body and soul.

Who Is Responsible Here?

This point leads directly to the second part of the responsibility, which is responsibility for health. The keys to healing are in our hands and not in the hands of any external factors such as my physician or my environment. In the first chapter, which discussed the reasons for the difficulty in listening to the soul, I noted that blaming the other is one of the most convenient, easy, cunning, and practical tactics we humans have developed for getting to feel better about ourselves, just like the tactic of disparaging the other in order to elevate ourselves. Both result in a momentary improvement of our self-perception, which leads immediately to a better feeling. And we all want to feel better, as much as possible and as quickly as possible.

In order to withstand the rigors of the path of healing and self-recovery, we must assume full responsibility for the process and end the habit of blaming our genes (I was born that way), our parents (they never encouraged me to succeed), our primary school teachers (that witch told me that I was stupid), our doctors (he said I couldn't succeed), our bosses (he constantly yells at me), our colleagues (I do everything and they do nothing), our children (I have no time for myself), or our neighbors (what is so bloody hard about closing the lid of the trash can?).

Blaming others leads us to focus ourselves on them, exactly the opposite of what we should be doing when we commit to self-healing. **Self-healing is all about focusing on yourself, the guiding principle being to maximize internal introspection and minimize external extroversion.** Obviously, we can't shut ourselves off from the world, and we all have a thousand and one commitments, tasks, and daily chores, but the overall goal is to minimize our involvement with others as much as possible and to expand our involvement with ourselves as much as possible; To define that as a target and see where it is possible and when it is possible. I do not mean narcissistic involvement or buying another pair of shoes to stuff into the overflowing closet. No, what I mean is a conscious choice to place oneself in a state of high attentiveness to oneself.

When Is the Responsibility for Recovery Expressed?

The responsibility for recovery is expressed on two occasions: when you choose to take the first step on the path of self-healing and when you fail to walk that path. Your path to self-healing is personal and will reveal itself as you walk it. You will be exposed to a great deal of advice from many professional parties from many different fields.

Not only will the various parties not always agree, they will often try to pull you toward the path they favor. (And again, it doesn't really matter if your path to healing is conventional or alternative-holistic. Each of these groups has quite a few possibilities and experts.)

When you approach the path of healing from a starting point of assuming responsibility, you are more attentive to which option feels right for you and most suits who you are. What is good for one person is not always suited to another. Each and every one of us is special and unique, and no one knows you better than you do.

What happens when you fail time and time again? First of all, you are disappointed. Then you try to find someone to blame. That is our default, automatic response. That is how we are used to behaving. We don't really control it, and particularly not when we have paid money to a professional and relied on them, or even pinned our hopes on them. When a treatment fails and we do not achieve the results we yearned for, we are frustrated and lash out. He is the one who is at fault; it his treatment that sucks.

When we take responsibility for our own path to healing, our failures teach us two important lessons. The first is that you need a great deal of patience to let the healing process succeed. There is no magic trick. Well, there is. Miracles have happened, do happen, and will happen, but you should not pin all your hopes on them if you do not wish to be disappointed.

Your chronic diseases were the work of many years, and they will not disappear overnight or after a single treatment. **They are chronic precisely because they symbolize something that is chronically imbalanced deep within us and change, as we well know, takes time. Changing habits takes the longest.** If I am used to flagellating myself at every opportunity, no miracle will cure that overnight. Patience for ourselves and for the healing process, which includes failures as well as successes, is required.

The second lesson is that perhaps this specific treatment is not right for us or for our bodies. It may have done wonders for other people who recommended it to us—that is why we chose it, after all—but it is not having the same effect on us, and that is just the way it is. There is nothing you can do about it. Well, nothing productive anyway. Feel free to complain, grouse, blame others, and even sink into despair for a while. It's okay. At some stage, whether an hour, day, or month later, we will rise, shake the dust off our clothes, and choose to continue, because by then we will remember why we set off to begin with.

The inner voice already knows it must remind us and guide us. The process of rising up becomes easier and shorter when we take full responsibility for the path we take and the choices we make along the way, even when the results are frustrating and disappointing.

RESPONSIBILITY IS AN ENGINE

It is important to stress this point that assuming responsibility for the disease will not, in and of itself, cure anyone. It isn't supposed to; that's not its job. Responsibility is the engine that motivates us forward and impels us to continue, just like our ego does (well, at least when we are able to control it and push it out of the driver's seat).

By choosing to assume responsibility, we are choosing to rely on our intuitions, we are choosing to listen to the wisdom of the inner voice that guides us and to be aware and attentive to it. We choose our own self.

But what do we do when our own self is no great shakes? What happens when I am not used to appreciating myself? What happens when I have low self-esteem or no self-esteem whatsoever, regardless of what led me to this extreme state? What happens when I appreciate and admire everyone around me but not myself? What happens when I feel foolish compared to all of the medical experts who have spent so many years mastering their craft? What if I don't think I can rely upon myself, or think it better to remain silent?

If you have no time, because you have been diagnosed with a terminal or severe disease, then you really have no choice—you will have to clear up your life and immediately become attentive to yourself, if you wish to increase the odds in your favor. Remember Rule #1: **No expert in the world knows what is best for YOU more than yourself, even if, up until now, you have done a crappy job in regard to self-attentiveness**.

The rules of the game have changed. That expert can recommend a course of action on the basis of his extensive experience, or maybe different experts will recommend a course of action, but only you can choose what is best for you from all of these alternate courses of action. Start relying on yourself, dare for once in your life to trust your judgment and to back it up. Assume responsibility and begin to study and investigate all of the options available to you. Learn from others who were in the same situation you were and made it. Get out of the paralyzing and fixating framework of "I don't know enough."

Assume responsibility, because there is no time, because the clock is ticking, because it is important to you, because you want to live. Where there is no time pressure and it is "only" a chronic disease or any other physiological phenomenon that requires pills and you feel it is hard for you to rely on yourself, start asking, investigating, consulting, listening, opening up, and daring to leave the space you are stuck in. **Assume responsibility for expanding your knowledge before you take any practical steps.**

It took me five years to make a decision to embark on the path of self-healing, in spite of not having any self-confidence issues or underappreciation of my intelligence. I studied and learned for five whole years, until I reached the point where I told myself that if others had made it, there was no reason in the world for me to fail. I studied up to the point where I dared to actually do something contrary to what the doctors had told me. I studied up to the point where I understood how much the doctors knew and don't know and the limiting constraints they operate under. I learned until I reached the point where I trusted myself, and from that point on, I assumed personal responsibility for my health, with maximum attentiveness to my intuitions.

Something nice and encouraging that happens when you assume responsibility is the disappearance of fear. "What will happen if I do not succeed?" disappears from the daily radar, and instead you feel the full power of the insight "I have created this disease and now I am creating health." This insight provides all the energy required to walk the new and unfamiliar path. Trust yourself to select the best options proposed for you.

When you assume responsibility, you suddenly see, very clearly, that no one else can really assume responsibility for our lives. The "others," as an overall term for all the doctors, healers, and caretakers out there, can't really assume responsibility for your life or your recovery. All they can do is offer you the best that they know and are experienced in, and they do. They can assume responsibility for the treatment itself, but none of them can assume responsibility for your life.

That's how this world works, and for a good reason we are the only ones who can and should assume responsibility for ourselves. So when we are finally at the point where we assume responsibility for ourselves, there is no need for anyone else to assume responsibility for our lives. We fulfill our role in the best possible way. We make our own choices.

To Summarize the Third Key

- Assuming responsibility for creating the disease is the understanding that part of us, mostly hurt and injured, created the disease, and that this is an unconscious process.
- When you undertake a commitment for self-healing, you must focus on yourself, not on blaming someone else.
- Responsibility for the healing process is expressed when we select the path of healing that is best for us.
- Our failures teach us that the healing process requires patience and that not every treatment is right for us and for our body.
- Personal responsibility is an engine that feeds off attentiveness to the self.

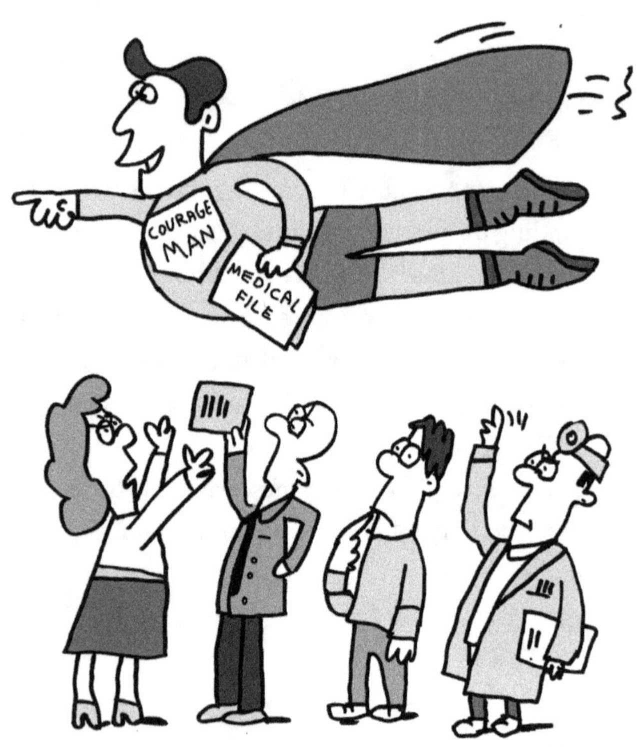

Self-healing is not for the faint of heart. Without courage, you probably cannot embark on the path, let alone complete it.

COURAGE TO EMBARK ON THE PATH

"Faith is taking the first step even when you don't see the whole staircase."

— Martin Luther King, Jr.

Self-healing is not for the faint of heart. Without courage, you probably cannot embark on the path, let alone complete it. This requires immense amounts of courage. Where can you acquire it? Excellent question. The answer is twofold: it either shows up on its own under extreme conditions or you need to produce it from within.

Some will say you either have courage or you don't. You are either brave or you aren't. You were born with it. Courage may flow from within. It is not beamed from external sources, but it is certainly possible, at any point in life, to plant seeds of courage and nurture them much as you cultivate a seedling—slowly but surely, at the proper and natural pace, with proper feeding, attention, and much patience.

There are some extreme conditions when the courage does arrive from nowhere, such as when the angel of death knocks on your door in the form of a severe or terminal illness, a heart attack, a stroke, or any type of extreme and challenging wake-up call. The courage just shows up one day, out of the basic instinct to survive, to live, out of the renewed recognition of the value of our threatened gift of life.

It doesn't really matter who you were until that wake-up call, until that ringing slap that led you to think your body had betrayed you. It doesn't really matter that you never had the courage to do things like you always saw people around you do. It doesn't matter that you never dared leave your comfort zone or never had the courage to say yes to challenging opportunities that passed you by, or never con-sidered yourself to be courageous. That wake-up call will usually rock your world sufficiently, including some of what you believe about yourself, to create a platform for radical and significant changes, including the appearance of the willingness to fight for your life.

But what happens when there is no immediate threat to your life? What happens where there is no external actor to deliver the wake-up call? Where do you bring the first seeds of courage to be planted and nurtured, assuming there is no plant nursery near you that has such magical seeds for sale?

What you do is reach a conscious decision that "I want to cultivate my courage, and I want to use that courage to embark on the path of self-healing." Don't underestimate the empowering force of making a decision and stating and knowing your true will. That is when you began to fertilize the ground with the inspiration you can get from others who were once where you are now. You read about them, you watch them on documentaries, you meet up with them—people who are the furthest thing from your image of courage-drenched warriors, just ordinary people whom extraordinary circumstances have forced to embark on incredible journeys.

Luckily, we live in an age where all this information, from all over the world, is just a click away. You don't even need to step out the door or get off the sofa to begin your journey. It's enough to access YouTube or ask on Facebook, "Who has heard? Who knows?" or even just raise the subject with a friend on the phone. Be certain that the information will flow in.

All you need during the first stage is to express your intention and willingness to be open to listening. During the second stage, you will initiate the process of inspiration and attentiveness (the fertilization), and slowly the seedling will bud out and emerge onto the surface. Slowly you will generate the courage to embark on your challenging inner voyage.

Many Uses for Courage

Why do we need courage? There are many uses for courage, and I will iterate a few of them. The first is that **courage is required to overcome the loneliness of the intensely personal path of self-healing,** a loneliness that scares quite a few people. There will be many contact points with various entities, professional or otherwise, but percentage-wise this makes up only a tiny part of your time.

Most of the time, you will be alone, and it won't be simple to walk the road alone. You will be alone because it isn't a team hike but **a personal journey deep into the depths of your soul and spirit.** You will be alone, but you won't be truly lonely because you will have yourself. The saying "If I am not for myself who will be for me?" is right on. You may find many good people on your road of self-healing, and on some level or another you will meet them or pass by them, but their roads are their own.

It takes courage to help ourselves. We all want to help ourselves, or at least we declare so publicly, but how many of us actually do something about it? How many of us pass the stage of talk and take action? How many of us get stuck in wanting to want? Helping ourselves makes us scared. Helping ourselves paralyzes us.

Am I even worthy of help?

No one ever helped me, so why should I help myself?

Who am I anyway?

Where does this presumption, this chutzpa, this arrogance, come from?

It takes courage to look in the mirror and see what we don't want to see, what we had suppressed in order not to see, what we had forgotten because it hurt to see.

It takes courage to face our demons, who have been lying silently in wait, with eternal patience for the moment we would open the deeper basement doors and let some light in.

It takes courage to hear the untold story of the soul. It takes courage to face off against dignified and learned professionals, some of them arrogant and insensitive, who will tell you the opposite, that it can't be done, and who will make you feel small. Very small. Perhaps even foolish.

It takes courage to face family and friends, who will tell you that you are bonkers, that you are nuts, that you are making a mess of things, that they really don't understand where you got these oddball ideas, that they are really disappointed with you, that you don't understand how many charlatans are out there, and that you could die playing these games, and they would never forgive themselves for it.

It takes courage to get up after a fall—and chances are that there will be falls. Unless you are one of the rare few for whom all will flow smoothly, you will stumble now and again. But since you have courage, you will know deep inside that at this point failure means nothing about the rest of the way, and you will rise, return to the main path, and carry on.

This Is Scary

Most people find it hard to accept this information. First, it frightens them because everything that is linked to death, whether directly or indirectly, is scary. **So long as we are cut off from our source, separated from it while living within a linear illusion of beginning, middle, and end ("For dust you are and to dust you will return"), we are**

in constant fear of extinction. That same fear of extinction contrasts with our most basic instinct here on Earth, preservation of the existence of matter. So it is better to suppress this troubling fear from our everyday life because there are enough other issues to deal with.

Second, the embarkation on your journey of self-healing provides a mirror to those around you that they really don't want to look into, or that they find hard to look into. If you stepped into their shoes, you would see that it isn't simple to watch someone close to you taking the steps that you would want to take given other circumstances, other times. or a different environment. They might say, "Right now, it is not possible" or "I can't afford this" or "I wish I had his courage." So there is no point in judging them. That is how people act, and you need to accept it.

Still, you don't have to share everything with everyone. **It is recommended that you apply a filter of information to the environment, in accordance with the level of support they provide, or conversely, the level of fear they display or the level of energy they are draining from you.** Often it will be better to provide your circle of friends and loved ones with general, optimistic information, such as "Everything is fine. I'm taking care of myself, and it will be all right," because the whole truth is complex and challenging, and not everyone can deal with it.

Permit yourself a little temporary egoism which, for you, means "I am in the center now. Only I matter right now. My mental and physical health is important, and all the rest less so." Right now, during the period of your recovery, you can allow yourself to be egotistical. You need every drop of energy you have to make this temporary journey.

It is not merely a lifestyle, not merely a "forever more," but also this moment is your time to help yourself. I promise that as soon as you are done helping yourself, you will automatically desire to help others. You will be able to pay it back. Right now, all of what you are needs to be focused toward yourself in order to depart, in the future, from a reinforced position, a connected, clean, whole, and healthy place.

So yes, there are children and significant others and commitments such as work, of course there are. We all have them and we must all face them, because it is unlikely that a genie will emerge from any nearby lamp to toss us off to a placid parallel universe that is absent of commitments and obligations where we can deal with ourselves. We must do this in parallel with life itself and therefore, beyond the absolutely minimum requirement, the rest can be shifted away temporarily. Beyond that bare minimum for which you are responsible, **don't waste any energy on those who will squeeze out your energy. Save it for yourself. You will need it at this period more than usual.**

SUPPORT, SUPPORT, SUPPORT

The only category of time and space worth expending your energy on is seeking supportive environments. Such an environment will support, empower, and fill up your reservoir for the journey to come. We are talking movies, books, supportive friends, or support groups—regular meetings with people who have already walked the path and those who are in the same situation you are. Don't underestimate the importance and power of such a support group.

Prevalence and consistency significantly alleviate all of the negative experiences you will run into along the way, and they also strengthen your faith. Your energetic reservoir will be filled and your courage will get a renewed boost as well, in each and every meeting, because there is no one as wise as the experienced person and because only someone who walks the exact same path as you do knows what sensations, emotions, and experiences, both negative and positive, you are going through. Everyone else can only guess or interfere, even if they have the best of intentions.

The additional and super-significant factor that fits into the supportive environment category is a professional and supportive team, headed by a "conventional-plus doctor"; in other words, a real doctor with additional therapeutic training. A doctor who is open to additional possibilities beyond those they have learned in medical school and beyond what the medical companies tell them under the "scientifically proven" excuse. This is a doctor who understands that the source of diseases is in the soul, and that in order to heal, one must treat the emotional-spiritual aspect as well as the physical one. **In other words, a doctor with a comprehensive holistic perspective.**

A supportive doctor can be the difference between

life and death. When a doctor tells someone that he has three months to live he is, for most people, pronouncing a death sentence. Very rare are the people who dare to challenge their doctor's judgment. Even if consciously they want to live, subconsciously they are preparing to die, because the doctor has told them they are going to die and the doctor must know what he is talking about.

Support from a professional, particularly from a doctor, constitutes a massive difference in general, and particularly in crisis moments when courage and motivation are low and there is no faith or vision. All there is is despair in large quantities, and a single word of encouragement from the doctor is sufficient to change the situation completely and reignite the spark.

This kind of doctor is not afraid to offer encouragement. This kind of doctor is not afraid to be optimistic. This kind of doctor has seen others like you walk down the path of self-healing, and may well have opened himself up to options beyond those taught in medical school after he himself recovered from a disease in a non-conventional manner.

Besides that doctor, you will have to recruit other professionals and caregivers of all sorts (nutritional, movement, mental, energetic, spiritual). Unfortunately, you are unlikely to find them in the standard hospitals or medical clinics, which means you will have to invest far more time and money in order to find them.

I recommend you view these expenses as an expression of confidence in yourself, in your abilities, and in your honest self-love. You will thank yourself for this gift each and every day you walk on this planet healthy and free of pills, because it will be worth every penny you spend. Believe me, I have nothing against fancy cars or clothes, a new pair of shoes, a vacation abroad, electronic gadgets, or other consumer goods. But how much more will you enjoy all those things when you are truly healthy and happy?

Do you have the courage to embark on this path? Do you have the courage to help yourself? Do you have the courage to change?

SUMMARY OF KEY NUMBER 4

- A great deal of courage is required to walk a lonely and highly personal road, to help ourselves, to look in the mirror, to face our demons, to stand up to professionals, family, and friends, and to get up after a fall or a failure.
- Sow the seeds of courage through receiving inspiration from others who have walked the same path.
- Don't waste energy on people who will drain you of energy; keep it for yourself.
- The importance of a supportive, non-judgmental environment, both personally and professionally, is immense.

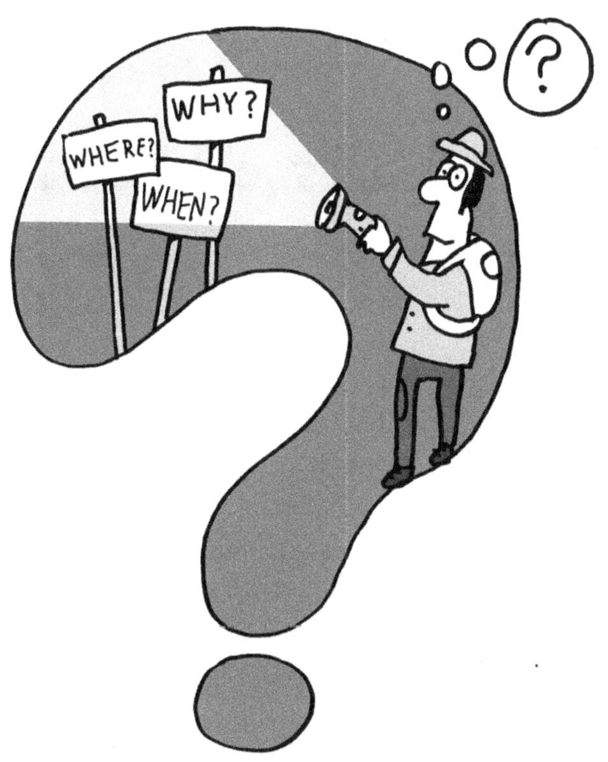

Self-healing is based on deep internal reflection, on the spring cleaning of quite a bit of emotional debris, and brave confrontation with your demons. This path encounters many, many questions.

KEY 5
QUESTIONS, QUESTIONS, QUESTIONS

If you wish to get well, regardless of your disease, prepare to ask yourself many tough questions. Self-healing is based on deep internal reflection, on a spring cleaning of quite a bit of emotional debris, and brave confrontation with your demons. This path brings up many, many questions. You won't always get answers to them either.

More accurately, the answers won't come immediately because they aren't even present in the conscious part of your brain. But the very fact that you put yourself in a place to ask questions is already advancing you one step at a time toward the longed-for recovery, since this indicates that you have chosen to be aware of yourself, aware of the situation, aware of the fact that the disease was created by a part of you, and also that you have assumed responsibility for it and know that you have the ability to get well.

The questions you should be asking are divided into two categories: the "what" questions and the "where"

questions. It is recommended, when you start out, to ask them with the support of a professional, whether a therapist or any other companion you choose to involve in the process, since the answers that emerge to these questions, at the wrong place and time, will not always be pleasant and easy to digest. It is therefore suggested that you place yourself in a supportive, accepting, helpful, and above all else, non-judgmental environment, because you will be judging yourself quite enough as it is.

So What Is It All About?

The first type of question is the "what" type. It is based on you accepting and internalizing the premise that your disease is the language in which your soul is speaking to you. **That is the premise you must accept to make this work.** You need to ask your questions from a courageous place that really desires to know the answers, regardless of what they are, to the following questions:

- What is the story that my soul is trying to tell me?
- What is it struggling with?
- Who or what hurt it?
- What have I forgotten that it is trying to remind me of?
- What issues have I suppressed that I must now deal with?
- What point in time did it try to reach me?
- What are the early signs that I ignored?
- What will soothe my soul?

What, that's it? Sounds way too simple, right? I promise you that "simple" is far from what this little research is. These questions constitute some of the most difficult obstacles you will ever face, and some of you will not even reach that point. Something internal will prevent you from asking these questions, precisely because of that inbuilt survival mechanism that protects us and guards us from getting hurt—hurt of the more serious, internal, emotional, invisible, non-tactile, inaudible kind. It can just be felt and it feels terrible, it feels so unpleasant.

And then, in order to return ourselves to a pleasant situation, we suppress it. We supposedly only hurt ourselves when we ask these questions and raise things that we have forgotten, but only supposedly and only temporarily. This still requires us to get over those parts that do not want to hear or remember the answers to these questions.

An extremely important study performed in an orphanage in Romania found **how acutely important love is for the sound development of children.** The study investigated the harsh and cruel reality that many children and infants who grew up in these orphanages received no audial (loving, comforting, soothing, encouraging words) or tactile (caressing, hugging, kissing) expressions of love. This terrible neglect harmed their development and created severe emotional and physiological problems for them later on.

Most of us did not grow up in an orphanage, but **how many of us never received sufficient encouragement or loving contact? This deficiency has consequences. Be sure of it.**

Two issues probably resonate in your mind while you are wondering if you are prepared to ask yourself these tough questions. The first is that **most people in the world have experiences in which they feel that they are not loved or they are worthless.** How exactly "I am worthless" is felt or reasoned is very personal. It may be expressed as "I don't know," "I don't understand," "I can't," "I am not managing to accomplish everything on time," "I am not worthy," "I do not deserve anything good," "I deserve to be beaten," "I don't deserve to be treated with respect," or a whole variety of other negative personal interpretations.

Our imaginations are limitless. All of us, or nearly all of us, deep inside, have these malignant thoughts in our minds that run our lives by making us respond, think, or feel differently than we might otherwise wish.

The second issue emphasizes that **the untold story of the soul need not be necessarily related to childhood, whether you have been hurt or abused, or whether you were insulted or humiliated.** There are more than enough other stories from other periods in life, including our adult lives. This includes severe trauma like a sexual assault or inability to deal with the loss of a loved one.

For example, it has been found that incidents of cancer among family members of the victims of the September 11 World Trade Center terror attack were dozens of percentage points higher than the national norm.[3] But it also includes lesser trauma such as a layoff, a hard divorce, too much stress over a prolonged period, unresolved inner conflict, lack of self-love, and low self-esteem (from "I don't deserve a promotion" to "I don't deserve respect" to "I don't deserve to live"), disappointment from God, and all sorts of other nuggets. We are complex creatures with quite a few confrontations we have to face in life. The question is, what do we choose to do about it?

Do we accept it as an act of God, or assume responsibility

---

3   I was exposed to this information in the lectures of Brandon Bays, creator of The Journey healing method. She was fortunate enough to have the opportunity to support and aid the families of the 9/11 victims.

and act for change by asking questions out of a real desire to face the answers head on out of a true desire to handle the answers once and for all?

LOCATION, LOCATION, LOCATION

The other type of question refers specifically to the location of the disease, and it emerges from the premise that there is enormous importance to the location of a disease in the body.[4] A good part of the healing process is mediated through finding an answer to the question "Why am I sick in this specific location?" What is the story of the afflicted organ? What does it represent? What is it responsible for? What is its role in the body? What passes through it? What does it represent for me?

It is important to note two things. The first is that **this is purely subjective interpretation. Each and every one of us has a prism through which we view life, analyze it, interpret it, and finally act according to it.** The meaning that one person gives to the word *heart* might be fundamentally different than that of another. For one, the heart symbolizes giving or compassion, while to the other it may symbolize hurt and heartbreak.

That is why you must take all the examples provided here and pass them through your own specific and unique

---

4   One of the first people to discuss this issue was Louis Hay, in her book *You Can Heal Your Life*.

filter. The second thing worth mentioning is that **the game we will play here with the organs and their significance is only the starting point in the search for the reason and source of the disease.** It is an excellent starting point that might form a significant shortcut, focus you specifically, and save you quite a few questions and inner conflicts, but it cannot spare you the need to walk the path itself, or the immersion into the source and primal cause of your woes. I will begin, if you will permit me, with the simplest organs, those that do not require a great deal of work to draw conclusions about because their defined roles are very clear.

Legs: The legs serve us to walk, to transition from place to place, to go forward. When a pain or disease shows up in your feet, ask yourself where you are stuck. Are you standing still? Where do you refuse to walk, progress, or move? Are you afraid of taking the next step?

Knees: The knees are the flexible part of the legs that bend. Where do you find it hard to bend and be flexible? What change or transition kindles unwillingness to change or be flexible? Where are you rigid and inflexible? Where is this rigidity attached to your progress or your refusal to move forward?

Eyes: The eyes represent our view of the world. What do you refuse to see about yourself or your environment? What is hard for you to see in the past, present, or future? In what field in life are you not in full focus? What do you blur out? Can you see what you are doing to yourself? Where are you unfocused? What have you seen that scares you?

Ears: The ears represent our ability to listen to the

world. What are you refusing to hear, either about yourself or others? What have you heard that fills you with rage or fear? What is hard for you to hear? Who do you refuse to listen to? Are you more attentive to outer sounds than to inner ones?

Throat: Your throat represents your ability for self-expression. Do you represent yourself? Do you dare express what is in your heart? Do you know how to ask? What do you dare not say? What have you wanted to say but have been forbidden to? What are you afraid to say?

Neck: Your neck represents your flexibility. When your neck is stiff, try to think what parts of your thinking are rigid. To whom do you express this rigidity? What situation extracts from you a stubbornness or lack of flexibility?

Back: The back represents our support system. and Where do you feel that you don't get support? Are you missing emotional, spiritual, or mental support? Who does not support you as you would like? Is there someone stuck behind you whom you refuse to see or can't see? Do you feel like you have been backstabbed? What burdens you the most? Where do you feel most overburdened?

Stomach: The stomach represents our ability to digest life in the form of our ideas, thoughts, or experiences. What is hard for you to digest or swallow? How do you digest reality? What is stuck and not flowing? What feels like a punch to your stomach? Our digestive tract can demonstrate to us that we are having a hard time absorbing reality, or that we can't keep pace with it so that things simply pass through us. Constipation indicates that we are holding things in, failing to express or execute them, so they all stay inside, stuck.

Heart: The heart represents (how unsurprising) love. When you deny yourself love, the heart cools and constricts. When you are surrounded by love, the heart warms up and expands. Where in your life is love lacking? What within you does not flow with love? Who is not giving you love, in the past or the present? Are you happy? Who is denying you love? Is your heart open or closed? Are you attentive to your heart

Breasts: Breasts represent, above all else, nurturing and motherhood. Where do you give too much? Is motherhood nullifying your selfhood? Are you demonstrating excessive maternity toward an individual or a place or an experience? Have you forgotten, because of your motherhood, how to receive? Do you remember what it is to love yourself? Do you know when to let go of your children and let them find their own way? What does the term "over-mothering" mean to you? What feelings does it raise?

Lungs: They represent our ability to breathe life in. Without breath, without oxygen, we could not live. Do you find it hard to contain life? Are you sufficiently connected to life? Do you have thoughts that life may not be worth living, that life is too harsh or the world is too cruel? Is someone or something sitting on your chest and making it difficult for you? Are you failing to let go of grief or regret? When and where do you feel it is too difficult for you to breathe? What is hard for you to let in, and what is hard for you to let out?

Skin: Our skin serves as a boundary layer between ourselves and the environment. Do you feel isolated from your environment? Or, alternately, do you feel that you have lost your uniqueness? Do you feel you have merged too much with other people? Is something, or someone, threatening your space? What is getting through your skin? Do you have a need to shout out your individuality? Are you crying out to be noticed?

Reproductive organs represent our masculinity or femininity. Are you okay with your sexuality? What do you feel toward your sexual organs? Do you accept them with love or view them as profane? Are you aware of them or do you repress them? Do you feel dirty when you engage in sexual activity? Do you cling to distorted beliefs about your body or its functions? What does the word *sex* make you feel? Do you feel a need to punish yourself after engaging in sexual intercourse?

If your illness is centered on an organ that you don't really understand, such as the spleen or the gall bladder, then open up Wikipedia and read about its functions. What is it responsible for? What functions does it fulfill? Try to reason from there how that might be related to your emotional experiences.

For example, the liver is a super-important organ that, among its other functions, is responsible for poison filtration. Ask yourself if you encounter toxins during your life. Are you in an environment that is emotionally toxic? Do you have a hard time excluding toxins or emotional waste?

This key is like a complex treasure hunt with many clues of different types scattered across the trail. The game requires a great deal of attentiveness, willpower, courage, honesty, imagination, and even vision in order to get answers to all of these questions, but your reward at the end of the trail is well worth it!

TO SUMMARIZE THE FIFTH KEY

- The questions you must ask are divided into two types: the "what" questions such as "What is the story I am being told?" and the "where" questions such as "Why do I hurt there?"
- Most of us have experiences of feeling unloved or worthless.
- The untold story of the soul need not be linked to childhood.
- The location of a disease is a starting point in the search for its source.
- Our interpretation of the significance of the location of a disease is personal and subjective.

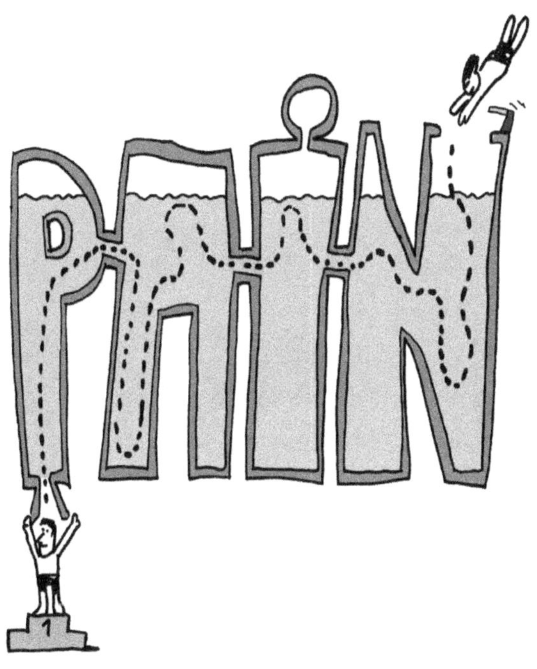

The path of self-healing is interwoven with pain. It is painful to release the congealed pain of the past, but this new pain has a purpose.

OUCH, IT HURTS!

"What kind of person chooses to feel pain? My God, just thinking about pain makes me feel queasy and stresses me out. So why should I venture into painful places? What good is all this pain?"

The pain I am talking about is the pain of emotional turmoil; it has nothing to do with physical pain. We are talking about "my heart aches," "my soul is in agony," and "I'm torn from within." This type of pain, my friends, hurts no less than physical pain.

Pain is a word that has frightened us ever since we were children. We are afraid of being hurt and so we do what we can, consciously or otherwise, to avoid pain, to flee pain, or to push it away as far as we can and as much as we can, whether by suppressing its causes in our minds or swallowing a pill to make the symptoms go away. Those who refuse to take pills we call masochists or just plain don't understand how their head works. Why do they choose to suffer? What sane person would choose agony over relief?

Those are reasonable, almost necessary, questions. The simplest way to answer them is by saying that **the pain has been within us for a long time already. Congealed pain, like a blood clot, deep within every cell of our body. The process of releasing that pain from our cells makes us feel it again. It hurts to release the pain. You might call the pain you feel during the release of the "old pain" the "new pain." This is a pain with purpose, a pain with a vision.**

This is the time and the place to make room in your heart for this pain and to remember that your soul has been in agony with the old pain for a long, long time. The fact that you do not feel it in your consciousness or in everyday life does not mean that your soul is not imprisoned down below where it is cold, dark, and lonely, twisting in agony, whimpering with pain, perhaps even wounded and bleeding.

WHY GO BACK?

"Why should I care?" you might ask. "It's done, it's over with, I have survived, and there is no going back." Seemingly, you are right. Still "I don't care, I'm not there anymore, I've moved on" is the answer of an individual who has closed their heart, an individual who has armored up their heart because they have been hurt in one way or another.

This is the time to shed your armor and dare to open up your heart, because you are actually opening

it up to an essential part of yourself. Even though others may have hurt you in the past, at the moment, only you can hurt yourself. You might ask, "Why not leave things as they are?" Well, you definitely could, but you will keep on being sick, continue to suffer, and continue to behave in a manner you don't really enjoy. You will have to continue to live with automatic thoughts, sensations, and responses that do not reflect your better side and which you cannot control. Why? Because all of these things are being transmitted to you from your soul. It is doing everything it can to get your attention; that is its language, that is what it knows how to do.

I did not invent these emotional human mechanisms. I am merely illuminating the path I myself walked down after listening to thousands of others who had walked down it before me and reached those same conclusions. **The road to self-healing passes through the gates of listening to your soul, listening to yourself, and loving yourself and all your aspects—and this road involves pain.**

"Reveal your shadows, or your shadows will reveal you."[5] This sentence transmits wisely, and deeply, the essence of the housecleaning we must perform. What are these shadows if not the darkened portions of the soul, our thoughts and emotions? There are deep-seated fears in there—shame, regret, judgments, injuries, and beliefs—which are blocking us from developing or accepting. We are less than proud of this part of us and don't want to present it to the rest of

---

5   I first heard this sentence from the spiritual teacher Teal Swan.

the world. But over time, if it is not listened to, this part of ourselves creates pain and diseases.

Yes, we are always told to think positively—to think positive thoughts and dwell on the positive—and then we will attract more positive things, right? Well, that is very true, and no one who told you this was lying to you. Still, this is not the whole reality.

Positive thoughts are not enough. Since the creator of our reality is our subconscious, it is that which is the real boss. Our subconscious is in control. Our consciousness is only responsible for a few percentage points of the party and so, for example, if we think all day "I want to live in plenty," but deep inside we believe that anyone who has a lot of money is corrupt or a crook—or alternately believe or think deep inside that we do not deserve to live in plenty— no great wealth will move our way, and even if it does, it will not remain long. How can it, when we subconsciously believe that we don't deserve it?

That is how the system operates. That is how affairs progress on this planet in the Homo sapiens department and in the self-healing realm. It is not sufficient to think positively in order to get well. It is not sufficient to say, "I want to get well" in order to become well. Nor is it sufficient to take a pill or change your nutrition or practice yoga in order to truly recover.

THREE ANALGESICS

After understanding why there is no alternative to feeling the pain, allow me to suggest three ways to ameliorate and dim it, if only partially. They will help you prepare yourself for the pain. It will still hurt, but less, much less. It will still hurt, but the pain will be tolerable, survivable.

The first way is to anticipate the pain. Anticipation reduces both the fear of the pain and the pain itself. You know the pain is coming. This is not an event out of your control or one that has caught you by surprise. You prepare for it, you are aiming at it, you mentally prepare yourself, and this creates an enormous difference in your attitude and how you deal with it, since you control the situation, even if only partially.

When we control a situation, something within us is more relaxed, less frightened, and less resistant to the situation. Deep within, you know that this is your creation, and so there is no need to be frightened of the pain when, or just before, it comes.

The second way is related to the temporal nature of the pain. Yes, it will hurt, but it won't hurt forever. Pain is merely temporary, because it is the pain of release. It might feel like forever, but it too shall pass. Just like on a cloudy day when everything is gray and disgusting and perhaps even cold and wet, the sun is still there above the clouds. It will always be there, even if we can't see it, and we will see it again as soon as the clouds scatter or move on their way, and we will be warm and comfortable again.

During those low points, the knowledge that the pain is temporary constitutes the faint flicker of hope and faith that it really will be okay and that you just need to let this pass, that this is part of the self-healing process.

The third approach refers to our free will, our agency, our choice. We chose this particular "new" pain over the "old" pain. We are transitioning from a state of escape to a state of choice. Unlike the past, where what happened was against us, or without our choice, we have been preparing for and intending to receive this new pain. The suffering might be terrible, but we choose to meet this painful place head on and consciously. We make the choice, and the power of such a freely made choice cannot be underestimated.

You can see its effects most clearly on children. When you let them make a choice, you get much more cooperation, even on tasks or chores they are not particularly fond of such as taking a shower or doing their homework. The choice gives them much more power over and control of the situation and therefore triggers less resistance and more cooperation.

This same mechanism works on us grownups. We chose this; it is our choice, no one made us do it, and no one forced it upon us. Therefore, we contain the situation better, we accept the situation more, and there is far less resistance to the situation, even when it hurts.

The darkness that arises from the depths is rising on its way out of your mind. Whatever emotions that you are feeling—be it anger, grief, fear, rage, depression, weakness, regret, guilt, or anxiety—and whatever pain you are feeling,

are rising up in order to release you, in order to cleanse you, in order to forgive, in order for you to move on and get well. You are more mature now than you were in the past, painful experience. You are more experienced, more certain, wiser, more accepting, more stable, more controlled, and have better analytical capabilities than you once had. All these will play in your favor at the moment of truth. Trust yourself. Your body and mind will be grateful to you and will express this gratitude in the form of health and happiness.

Don't fight the pain, accept it. It is here because you let it in, because it is its time to be released and to leave you. The pains and emotions are here because they are part of your healing process and serve your greater good. Trust them. Trust yourself. Trust the inner wisdom of your body. Trust your intuitions. Trust all of the preparatory work you have done prior to embarking on your way and everything you have learned from all those who have walked the path before you. **Trust in your pain. It is precise and anything but random. Nothing happens by chance.**

The process will walk you through a type of purification and cleansing. At its conclusion, you will emerge connected, empowered, and balanced—but this time, without any medication. Much like the conclusion of the movie *The Shawshank Redemption*, where the hero emerges from prison through the sewers, you have to swim through a lot of shit to break free. But break free you shall.

The Sixth Key Summary

- Letting go of your old pain will hurt.
- The "new" pain you feel during the release of the "old" pain is pain with a purpose.
- Anticipation of the pain reduces both the fear of the pain and the pain itself.
- The pain of release is only temporary.
- We transition from a state of escape to a state of choice.
- What rises does so in order to leave, in order to allow us to progress.

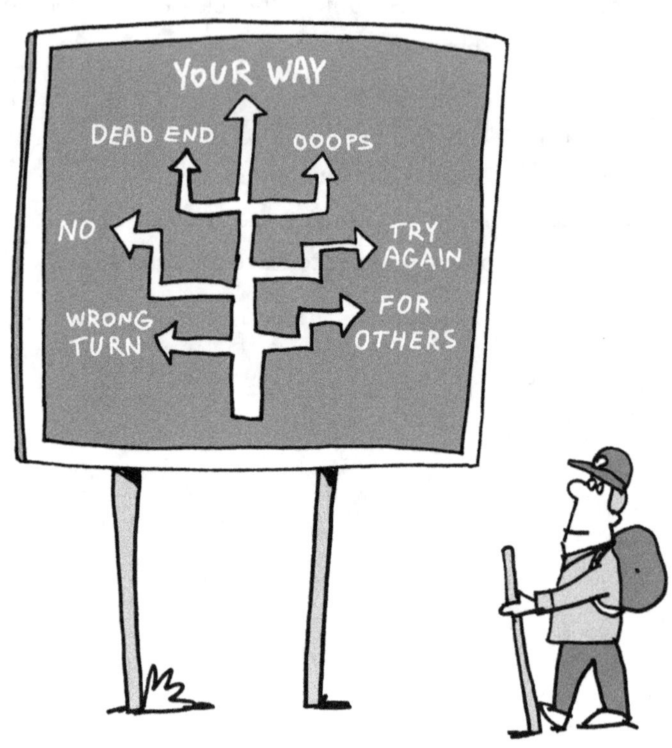

Every disease and every individual are a couple with their own specific path to recovery. No one path and no one solution fits them all.

EACH INDIVIDUAL WALKS A DIFFERENT PATH

Every disease-individual "couple" has their own specific way to get well. No path suits all people. There is no enabled copy and paste function. I mean, you can copy the document and paste it into your life, but humans are rather more messy and complicated than computers, and our manufacturer did not produce us from a single standard mold, so the results are unlikely to be what fits your needs.

Each of us has our own body, temporal soul, eternal spirit, different life story, other prisms through which we see and experience the world, different belief systems, and even other traumas, so there is absolutely no point in emulating my recovery story or that of anyone else. Nor is there any point in seeking to exactly emulate the treatments I or they underwent, regardless of how special or awe-inspiring you might find them to be.

What you can do is receive inspiration, courage, and energy from them to go out and discover your own personal path, one that will match you and your disease like a tailor-made glove. Our world has several channels of therapy.

(The four main channels are physical, emotional-mental, energetic, and spiritual.)But every therapy channel includes within it dozens of options. If we imagine the therapy channel as a highway, then we get many parallel roads and exits to side routes that all lead to the same place, just through different roads.

Each and every one of you has the unique combination that fits you and your disease. Just as none of the seven billion fingerprints on Earth are identical to one another, so does each individual/soul/spirit have a unique treatment regimen that fits it, and it alone, in accordance to the lessons we are meant to experience in this world.

There are diseases for which a single channel of treatment will provide you with a cure, and the problem will pass, possibly forever. Other diseases require a number of treatment channels, and some diseases require all of the treatment channels, particularly when it comes to chronic diseases that exist in our body over a prolonged period of time, as was the case with some of my diseases.

You cannot know in advance what will work and what won't work or where you will experience success and failure. That is why it is so important to embark on your path when you are prepared. That means seeking knowledge, being open to things that you do not yet know, having the courage to face whatever emerges from the depths of your soul, and maintaining a strong desire to recover and live a healthy life.

I will start with the more familiar channels, those that the most has been written about, and those easiest for you to swallow: the physical and the emotional-mental. Then we will transition to the two more escoteric and harder-to-digest channels for rational people: the energetic and the spiritual.

THE PHYSICAL CHANNEL

This channel is a world in and of itself. It is the most "scientifically proven" channel of the four, the only one that our five senses can perceive. It can be seen, heard, touched, smelled, or even eaten, which is why it is the most investigated, studied, and information-rich channel, sometimes to the exclusion of all others.

Should I describe the problem with this channel? Most of us already know all the information here, but we don't implement it in the field. We keep on looking for new magic solutions, new inventions that will provide instant cures and get us to the perfect place we want to be in regard to our looks, our weight, our behavior, our work environment, our living environment, or our self-perception.

The basic principle is invariable—the way we treat ourselves is the source of all diseases. Consumption of junk food and self-hatred are the basis of disease creation. No one ever taught this principle to us and even when we do learn it, it is still not at all easy to change habits, beliefs, or thoughts or open ourselves up to any type of change. That is why disease is a great opportunity to channel our energies into the new consciousness, with self-compassion and self-forgiveness, and use the disease as a lever to transform our lives and cure ourselves.

NUTRITION

The category that takes up the lion's share of this channel is, of course, our nutrition. Nutrition as a lifestyle, nutrition out of awareness of the negative effects of processed industrial food on our health, **nutrition as an opportunity to prove to ourselves that we truly love ourselves, an opportunity that passes directly through our stomachs and bowels.**

There are, seemingly, three "problems" with proper nutrition. The first is that if you do not suffer from excessive weight—in other words, if you approached the change in nutrition from a health-based rather than weight-based orientation—**you will not feel any day-to-day difference.**

If you are encouraged to add more vegetables and legumes to your diet and cut back on white flour and white sugar, you are not going to get up one day and feel completely different. It generally doesn't work that way with nutrition. There are certainly people who are more sensitive and notice small changes in sensations following the change in their diets, but I would not, if I were you, depend on that because you will just be disappointed.

This is exactly what happened to me, and it really frustrated and annoyed me. I had no proof that what I was doing nutritionally was the right thing, no indication to hold onto beyond the knowledge that I was providing my body with the building blocks it required for an optimal and sound function, including the specific foods that would help it in its process of purification and healing. (Vegetables, for example, can detoxify your body.)

The second problem is that proper nutrition takes time and has no immediate outcome, as is the case when one takes pain medication and the symptoms are immediately alleviated. **Nutrition is a long-term solution for a long-term problem, and it takes time before results can be seen.** Nonetheless, a painkiller might provide immediate relief, but is only a short-term solution with a very brief impact. Once it is flushed out of your system by the body, the pain will just show up again.

The purpose of proper nutrition is to prevent the return of pain and disease back into our lives, and a positive side effect is to keep us from developing new illnesses. As a result of the proper nutrition, your immune system will be toughened up, and do you know what happens to your immune system when it toughens up? It does its job the best possible way it can, and efficiently destroys whatever tried to harm you, no matter how minuscule it might be.

The third problem with proper nutrition, as of the twenty-first century, is information overload. There are already so many books, methods, recommendations, and techniques that tell you how to eat, what to eat, when to eat, and whom to eat with that some of us are already lost, especially since many of the methods contradict each other.

So which one is right? After all, each of these methods have been tested by people who managed to lose weight with them. (Unfortunately, in our society, the success of nutritional methods is defined by weight. Overall health is secondary.) So they all work. But which one is right? Which one should be chosen? Which one will best advance me in my goal of getting healthy?

My recommendation is to schedule an appointment with a professional who specializes in nutrition, who can adapt, for your specific body, a combination of blood tests, vitamins, and hormones, and a food cocktail that is most suitable for your specific body condition.

In my humble opinion, no method is a perfect fit for everyone. The neural system of someone who lives in a pastoral village is not the same as the neural system of someone who lives in a teeming city, and likewise for a person who lives in peaceful New Zealand compared to one who lives in conflict-plagued Israel, or someone who lives in a traditional society compared to one who lives in a competitive society filled with stress and pressure. Each of these factors has significant impact.

The first individual might have a severe deficiency in a given vitamin, which leads to certain problems in their system, while the other has different deficiencies that impact other systems, which is why a personal match is required. This also shows us how committed we are to ourselves and our healing processes, both now and during the paths we must walk until we return our souls to our creator, hopefully with a grateful smile.

Toxins, Out!

From nutrition, let us leap to non-nutrition, to the healing method that nature created—fasting. When animals are ill, they fast. When people are ill, they automatically experience a decline in their appetites. Even as babies, when we were ill, we had no appetite, and likewise when we were children.

Is this coincidence? Absolutely not, this is a feature, not a defect. When a person is ill, their immune system is occupied with fighting the infection. This war is the body's top priority, and it requires energy. What happens when an individual is not ill? What does the fast contribute to a body that is not engaged in fighting bacteria, viruses, or other invaders? The fast is an opportunity for it to carry out a detox, an internal cleansing of various types of toxins and waste that are stuck in the body, since the body does not know how to get rid of them. We are speaking here about toxins entering our bodies from environmental contamination, radiation, chemicals inserted into industrialized foods, chemicals added to our water, chemical fertilizers and contaminants inserted into the ground where we grow our food, drugs injected into the animals we eat and milk, and all of the hundreds of medications, hormones, steroids, and antibiotics we have received throughout our lives. All of them have a decisive impact on the quality of our functions and our immune systems.

When we fast, the body utilizes all of its available energy to carry out a thorough spring cleaning. The release of these toxins is expressed as headaches, skin rashes, weakness, or dizziness that pass after a day or two. Since a fast based solely on water is very difficult, it is easier to perform a juice fast. In a juice fast, filtered juices of vegetables and fruits containing high concentrations of vitamins and minerals required by our body are ingested several times each day. Accordingly, not only is there no sensation of fatigue, but most people experience a rise in vitality, joy, and energy levels. The fast increases the vitality of our physical and mental systems.

As long as we are discussing detoxing, allow me to share several steps I took along the way that I know played an important part in my recovery. The first is liver purification, which is intended to clean up all the poisons accumulated in the liver over the years (due to its role as a poison filter). In contrast to a juice fast, it does not require any special preparation or a total change in lifestyle, although it includes a five-day preparatory process and another two days for the purge itself. It is relatively easy to implement, and anyone can perform it at home. The protocol detailing the procedure is available online.

At the conclusion of this week, I had dozens of fluorescent-green spheres leave my body. Just the thought of them being in my body, in my liver, freaked me out. They did not look like something natural that should be in the body to begin with. I repeated the procedure three times over the year, and I am convinced that the physical purge played a major part in returning my body to a state of balance.

In addition, I regularly perform a hydrocolonic or hydrotherapy treatment, or an enema, to use the more common term. My colon is rinsed with a special instrument and an important part of the digestive tract is therefore cleansed, so wastes, some of which can be toxic, are expelled from my body.

What Else?

Additional physical channels we all know but find hard to implement on an ongoing basis because we can't find the time or wonder "What good will it really do?" include the following.

Breathing: We do not breathe well; our breaths are extremely shallow and rapid. Our bodies need us to breathe fully and deeply. It requires this oxygen like plants require sunlight. There are several contemporary therapy methods that teach people how to breathe, and there are amazing stories, including case studies documented by doctors who have studied the issue of oxygen as a healing method, that might cause you to rethink how you breathe.

In the regular course of day-to-day living, we do not stop to think about our breathing, because it is automatic, but we can try to adapt new habits to enable us to remember to breathe properly. **For example, remind yourself to take three deep breaths every time you sit in your car or on the bus. Every time you go to the restroom, remember, throughout your entire stay, to breathe slowly.** It doesn't really matter where or how much you breathe; the important thing is to pump your body full of oxygen. Oxygen can only improve your systems.

Water: Over 70 percent of our bodies are made up of water. We are, in fact, **walking bags of water. All of our systems function better when we drink sufficient amounts; conversely, our bodies function less efficiently when they are deprived of water.**

Any beverage containing sugar, food (fruit parts for example), chemical substances, or milk is not water. The body treats sweetened beverages like food, and does not fully utilize the water in that beverage. **Drink water for your health. If you do so meticulously, you will find yourself scrounging for far less junk. Often, we mistakenly interpret the body's thirst as hunger.**

Sun: Even those of us who live in semi-arid or subtropical climates often have a serious deficiency of vitamin C. The situation is even worse in the northern climes. It seems we are almost afraid of the sun since ozone layer depletion became an issue. But even though, unlike plants, we do not directly metabolize the sun's energy, we need it to initiate various biochemical reactions in our bodies, such as transforming cholesterol on our skin to the critical vitamin C.

So yes, while we do need to expose ourselves to the sun carefully and only during hours when it does not fry us like chicken, it is healthier for us, our physiological functions, and even our souls to put on a hat or a shirt to protect ourselves from the sun's rays rather than smear ourselves with various creams and ointments, or bar ourselves indoors. Nature, after all, created a fairly simple mechanism that is designed to identify when we have overdone exposure to the sun. "Are you sunburnt? Turning red? Then you are overdoing it—chill." I invite you all to look into this issue more deeply.

There are many books dealing with healing through controlled exposure to the sun. Yes, I am afraid that here too we have been indoctrinated into buying into a dogmatic equation of sun = danger = skin cancer. This equation is not true, and you have an opportunity to deepen your knowledge and win back the sun and all of its many advantages. **Look around you, at all of the living and growing things in our world. Everyone needs the sun, ourselves included.**

Sport: Yes, sport. Some people shudder when they hear this word, so you can use the term motion if you prefer. **The body needs to be in motion, because motion drives all systems in the body and strengthens your immune system. The key is to find the type of motion you most enjoy doing.**

You don't need a gym or a treadmill, which many among us view as severe punishment. Seek a motion-based activity that you enjoy, that you are good at, that you look forward to. Different styles of dance, walking with a good friend, bicycle riding, hopping on the children's trampoline, martial arts, or bouldering are all good. It doesn't really matter what you do, so long as you move your body.

It is true that sometimes it is simpler to suffer from your disease than to make a real effort at recovery, but if that is what you do, you won't maximize your chances of making a recovery. You need to approach the physical activity not from a place of "I need to do this," but from a place of **"I want to help my body recover. I want to live a healthy life."** Not from a place of "I need to lose weight," but from a place of **"I enjoy what I am doing."** If you don't do this, you won't be able to persevere, and that is a shame. Perseverance is hard for all of us. Always. That is why it is always better to alleviate where you can.

The Emotional-mental Channel

So how do you listen to your soul? What do you do in practice? You lie down on the therapist's sofa, you talk about it, you share, and then you heal? Probably not, because the fact is, quite a few of us lie down on the shrink's couch—it's no longer a badge of shame but a status symbol—but does that make our health conditions any better? Not really. For the most part, there is no connection between our health conditions and our mental conditions.

How does the average conversation with the shrink go?

"Why are you here?"

"I am unhappy."

"Why are you unhappy?"

Then you describe why you are unhappy.

Dozens of hours of complaints and belly-aching, some justified and some less so, follow. Now try to imagine for a moment what would happen if the starting point of your psychological therapy were different, if your starting point were initiated like this.

"Tell me why you are here."

"I am here because I want to assume responsibility over my disease. I am here because I choose to finally hear the story my disease is trying to tell me, and to thereby heal myself."

Think about this sentence as the starting point. Imagine that this is the first sentence you say in therapy. Think what that would do to and for you, and what that would do for your therapist. All of your therapy would flow in a different direction, one that is far better for the path of self-healing you chose to walk on. Yes, the pressure of life will flow into the therapeutic sequence, but **the starting point is different and is interwoven as a narrative throughout the entire therapy process, by seeking the emotional source of the initiation of the disease.**

Believe me, that source is there, quietly waiting for you, in the dark, for the moment you will be prepared to deal with it. The disease was created in order for you to reach this spot, where you speak about it, express your pent-up emotions (yell, scream, shout, weep, and lash out in your imagination), express yourself just as you always wanted to, cry out a bit more, and then release that source.

How do you let go? With the twin emotions of **thankfulness and forgiveness. Both have the ability to release us from our emotional prisons, the prisons of hatred and resentment we inadvertently place ourselves in. Both return us to the here and now and neutralize the effects of the past on our present.**

Thankfulness, like forgiveness, first releases the person who expresses it. It breaks down the bars. Hatred locks us in a small prison cell of self-pity, and releasing the past through forgiveness and thankfulness releases the present to be what it can be, what we want it to be.

Forgive not because the person who hurt you deserves forgiveness, but because forgiveness is the key to releasing you from your cell. Forgive straight from your heart. Don't say, "I forgive you" but continue to plan how to strangle the person to death or fantasize about rabid dogs breaking into their home and devouring them alive. Forgive fully, from the bottom of your heart. Forgive because that will release a great deal of energy that has been wasted on hatred and anger, which have mostly been self-directed. Forgive because it will make you better. **Forgive because it is simply time to move on.**

Our feelings are killing us, but they really don't have to, especially not when you have awareness and willingness, openness, and motivation to change things, even if what led you to this place was a disease. **Remember, the way forward is through your past. There are no shortcuts.**

A word about your therapist: You really don't need to see a psychologist with a formal education and qualifications. That isn't mandatory. Any therapist, from any field, with whom you have good chemistry, who generates good energy during your meeting, who you find pleasant to be around, who understands you, who provides good guidance, who is prepared to walk the road of self-discovery of the story of your soul as a stage in your recovery, and who supports you and your quest for health, can fit.

Trust your instincts. Ask friends for recommendations and then, **in the meeting itself, trust your feelings and sensations. Trust your heart. Does it warm up when you are with your therapist? The answer to that question is far more important than the type of certificate they have on the wall.**

Another recommendation is to **record your conversations with the professionals who treat you.** Do so for several reasons. First, so that you can hear yourself from a different perspective. This has an enormous impact. **You can learn a great deal from listening to yourself:** how you talk, how you respond, what you say, and how you sound.

Second, **you can catch up on things you might have missed during the meeting** because your mind was wandering or you might have lost focus occasionally. You might have missed crucial points.

Third, there is always a difference between hearing things days later, when you might be more relaxed, than at the session itself. **Perhaps you might even gain a few insights between the sessions with repeat listening, and thereby gain a type of a second session for the same price.**

Finally, you might want another person to listen to the words spoken in that meeting. You might have misunderstood or misinterpreted the session, and you can always use the assistance of someone else you trust by letting them hear the session or a portion of it. **You will thereby be exposed to another interpretation of the events, a more objective one, and profit by it.**

I have never run into a professional who refused my request to record our sessions, since this was always performed openly and was intended to optimize the therapy for which I paid good money. So don't feel bad or uncomfortable. It is legitimate and demonstrates your commitment to yourself and to the process as a whole.

The Energetic Channel

We have reached the two channels that challenge our pattern of thought, those who take us out of the ordinary, the known, and the revealed, but still have the potential to leave us gape-mouthed and scalp-scratching, not quite sure what happened or how the hell it happened.

When you say the word *energy*, many people start vibrating (which is funny, because we all vibrate all the time but are unaware of it), because they "don't believe in that nonsense" or think "there is no such thing" or because it is "completely speculative and unproven."

There are so many things in our universe that are irrational and inconceivable, starting with the basic building block of matter—from the atoms and all the particles and forces applied to keep them in the exact structure and configuration they occupy to the fact that life developed and that we live on a planet whose core is molten lava to the truly insane structure of the infinite cosmos.

And yet, the fact that energy flows through our bodies and that this energy can be used to heal is a fact we have a hard time grasping and accepting. It is with that fact, out of all others, that we suddenly develop issues of disbelief, and the absurdity is that we are not even alien to this energy. We feel it all the time.

Have you ever entered a room without knowing what happened between the people who were there before you entered, whether those present were a couple or business colleagues, and immediately felt tension so thick it could be cut with a knife? That tension is energy.

Have you ever entered the home of acquaintances, or even total strangers, and immediately felt as comfortable and pleasant as you do in your own home? When we speak of a pleasant atmosphere, we are talking precisely about the energy flowing in the home, and that energy primarily comes from the people living there. We can feel that energy at the level of our sensations.

When you are near an angry person, even if they are silent and say nothing, are your sensations pleasant? Do you feel calm or stressed out? Those are the energies they emit and you are responding to them. When you are near an adult, does it feel the same as when you are near a child? Are their energies identical? When you are vacationing in a cabin in the middle of the woods, are the sensations you feel the same as when you are in the city? When you are in the center of a desert or on a beach, the vibrations are totally different. The energy in nature is totally different, and that is when we feel the most sublime, the most connected to the universe, the most awestruck by the wonder of creation, and the most calm and relaxed. This is not by chance.

Everything in the Universe Is Energy

This energy is expressed or perceived by us in two ways. The first is life energy (called *chi* by the Chinese and *prana* by the Indians). This energy has no scientific proof. The second is the energy contained in all matter. This physical aspect of energy is scientifically established. (E = MC2, remember?)

Let's start with the physics. When you descend in matter to the level of basic components from which matter is constructed, you can see that the molecules of matter are made up of atoms, and that each atom is made up of different particles as well. At the center of the atom is the core, made up of high-mass energy particles called protons and neutrons. Revolving around this core are electrons, who orbit it at relatively high speeds. In other words, most of the atom is empty space.

The important thing is that the atom itself vibrates. Imagine a type of a vibrating energy ball connected to another ball of vibrating energy to form molecules, which also vibrate. These molecules form the building blocks of matter—matter that is made up, when you come right down to it, of vibrating energy.

Everything in our physical world vibrates in a unique frequency, including us humans. If we understand that all matter is actually energy, we need to understand that we too, in our human forms, are beings who vibrate in our own unique frequencies. Our environment's frequency has a positive or negative effect on us, depending on the frequencies that exist within us.

Now let's connected those dots together to life energy. **Life energy is the power that makes life possible.** It is what allows plants and animals to exist. It is what transforms a tiny seed into a massive tree, and it is what makes a sperm cell that comes into contact with an ovum into a whole and complex human body.

What happens to our body immediately after death? The life energy that flowed through it leaves it. **A human body without life energy is no more than organic, biodegradable waste.** "From dust you came, and to the dust you shall return."

In Chinese medicine, and in other ancient healing systems that have existed for thousands of years, this energy is treated with great respect. Every living and growing being contains within it different systems in which the constant flow of life energy occurs. **The energy flows through the body in channels called meridians, and each body seeks an energy flow that is as balanced and barrier-free as possible. Where blockages in the energetic body occur, they are expressed in the physical body in the form of pains or diseases.**

In the not-too-distant past, a German–Jewish scientist and psychiatrist named William Reich, studied, measured, and reached the same conclusion as the Chinese—**a universal life energy exists in dormant matter, plant life, every living life, and in the whole body.** His field of study included physics, engineering, sociology, psychiatry, and sexology.

Reich claimed that **the deficiency or injury to these life energies results in physical and psychological problems in human beings, and that restoring these energy fields solves these problems and makes possible a life of happiness and health.** Reich developed instruments to collect this energy and used them to cure various illnesses, including cancer. But the story did not end well. His research was confiscated by the government of the United States, and he was placed in prison, where he died of a heart attack.

WE DON'T KNOW WHAT WE STILL DO NOT KNOW

Each and every one of us must make a decision. Do we only heed and act upon what is scientifically proven? But before we reach that decision, we must consider this conflict. On the one hand, our glorious science studies the laws of nature, investigates everything we perceive in our reality, from the smallest micro cosmos to the largest macro cosmos. On the other hand, science has also found that nearly 90 percent of the matter that exists in our universe is invisible, and no one has the slightest idea what it is. That is why it is called "dark matter." It can't be seen, heard, smelled, or felt in any way we know, yet it still makes up the main part of everything that exists, including all the planets and galaxies in the cosmos.

We—the visible matter, the mass—make up 16 percent of the universe. The invisible dark matter makes up 84 percent of the universe. So what can we conclude from this? That everything that is scientifically proven is actually proven on only 16 percent of all that exists, and only on what we perceive to exist. We ignore 84 percent of the universe, because we do not know what is going on there, yet we allow ourselves to derive conclusions from that 16 percent and apply them to all 100 percent.

We do not know what we do not yet know, but not knowing it does not mean it does not exist. Once, it was "known" that the Earth was flat. Once, it was "known" that the sun revolved around the Earth. It was not only known, but those who dared to say otherwise or who tried to offer alternative explanations of the universe were burned at the stake.

Therefore, if we go back to the field of self-healing and the channel of energy therapy, **we can summarize that most of these types of therapy science have not yet been proven or investigated. Partially because those who have the money to study them are not interested in studying them, and partially because it is simply not time for humanity for to discover some things,** for reasons that the creator of the grand design we call existence is keeping to himself for now.

Still, you can permit your sensations to lead you while you hear of, and investigate, the myriad energetic therapy channels, while you experience them, hear of the experience of others, and just as importantly, **consider whether the therapy you selected helps you. Does it improve or relieve your condition or not?**

Each and every one of us has our own path of self-healing to walk, and each of us will discover the path intended for us one step at a time. Acupuncture or reflexology will perform wonders on one, whereas a second will use healing or reiki to release traumas imprisoned in the body. A third will undergo bio-orgonomic treatment to open up blockages and clean up their energy field. A fourth will call upon the angels for aid. And a fifth will reach energetic healing through aliens. (Yes, there is such a thing. People get well that way.)

There is even horse-based energetic healing. (Yes, that too exists. People are healed that way as well.)

Sometimes it is worthwhile to allow our mind to rest and allow our heart and sensations to take charge and lead us on, especially on a journey that shows us repeatedly that not everything we once knew is true.

The Spiritual Channel

If you found the energetic channel to be challenging, I am sure that the spiritual channel will be even harder. It is hard for us to accept things when we do not understand the mechanism they operate in. We find it hard to deal with things our mind can't compartmentalize. We find it hard to accept things that contradict what we have been taught and what we believe.

What is spirituality? Is spirituality prayer? Prayer to whom? If there were someone up there, he wouldn't abandon me and force me to go through all the suffering I am going through. Is spirituality meditating? I don't have the patience to sit still for half an hour; it is incredibly dull. Does spirituality require me to wear bell-bottom pants or robes, to stop shampooing my hair and to start growing dreadlocks, or to put feathers in my hair? Is spirituality being in love? Is spirituality chanting "We are one"?

There is no unity, everyone is out for number one, and people steal from, curse at, murder, humiliate, and harm each other daily. You need do nothing more than watch the news—

any edition will do, in any country, state, or territory—to get rock-solid proof of that. Well, that is certainly how things seem on the surface.

Still, as you read in the previous chapter, there are many things that we do not know and cannot see. Most occurrences take place beneath the surface or outside the range of our sensory perception. So put aside for a moment, just for a few minutes, what you know and the patterns you recognize, and try to understand reality from another perspective that is less rational and certain, and more intuitive and multisensory. Let things resonate within you and see what comes up. Once you are done reading, you can always say, "Hogwash!" and go back to being pissed at the world.

Is that enough preparation for the spiritual channel? Yes? Let's get started then. The meaning of the word *spirit* in ancient Hebrew (*ruach*) was "movement." Spirituality means the bidirectional movement of data from our material part, including the thoughts and emotions that are part of our temporal body and soul, to our eternal spiritual part, the supernal self, the divine spark.

This is the part from which arises our inspirations, unusual ideas, intuitions about people, places, or situations, gut instincts, and deep knowledge that bypasses our minds. "I knew from the very first second she would be my wife," "I knew I had to go there," or "Suddenly, I knew I had to study this profession."

Our two parts carry on ongoing communications with one another. The information passes from top to bottom and from bottom to top, and is cross-refer-

enced and processed in accordance to the master plan, according to our destinies and our roles, to promote the lessons we have come here to learn and to realize the highest potential of ourselves.

What is important to understand is that this communication occurs whether we are aware of it or not. Most of us are either unaware of it or don't know what to actually do with it, whereas others are aware of it but fear it.

SILENCE PLEASE!

Our supernal part does not dictate events or our actions, but it does direct them, since it is the part that is aware of our master plan and our role in the world. In our daily lives, it provides us with little clues that point us down the right track. Usually, however, we do not notice or hear them. Why? Because the world we live in is filled with noise and chaos, and we are bombarded at any given moment with infinite data, and also because **our supernal part speaks in whispers, not shouts.** They are very difficult to pick up, which is why in order to listen to both our temporal soul and our supernal, eternal spirit, we must be quiet. That is why we need to create a silent environment that will support the silencing of the external noises that drain away our attention and will enable us to listen to our inner voices.

That is the real point of meditation—temporary silencing of our systems so that we can listen to ourselves and receive information from our higher part. You don't have to assume the lotus position on the floor to do that; you can meditate while working in the garden, washing the car or the dishes, folding the laundry, jogging, painting, or sculpting.

Have you ever wondered why ideas and insights often appear when you are in the restroom or the shower? They occur because we are so focused on one thing that it creates a rare silencing of all other noises and thoughts. When it is silent, it is easier for us to pick up and hear the clues, messages, and directions that our supernal selves pass on to us in accordance to conditions on the ground and data received from our material selves.

Since it is not easy for most of us to begin practicing meditation—it takes time, training, faith, and dedication—we can begin by asking questions, by being aware. Most of us are comatose in regard to ourselves. Around the age of thirty, we tend to fall asleep each night thinking about the mortgage and the kids, and then find it harder to wake up and listen to ourselves.

Self-awareness is a first and necessary stage of wakefulness, because when you are awake, you begin to ask questions, and when you ask questions, answers begin to show up. All you need to do is aim the antenna and pick up the broadcast. To listen. That will begin to let us control our fates, to take control of ourselves, to move on from the victim phase where "life is happening and I have no control over it" to "I have greater control over things, understand why they happen, and am even learning from them." It is true that spirituality is not a free pass to the perfect life, but it has power and resilience that many of us are lacking.

In parallel, it is recommended that you employ the aid of therapists or spiritual teachers and channelers. They will help you by forming the connection between your supernal part and your spiritual guide, a sentient energy that knows you and accompanies you on the journey, knows everything about you, and seeks to transmit information that will aid in your development.

This therapy channel can transmit the information to you that you so desperately need in order to recover, such as an indication of the sources of your diseases. You might receive information regarding the tools that are practical for you to achieve your goals and fulfill yourself on the highest level. You can certainly refer to your connection to a spiritual guide as a rare and significant shortcut. It is super-important, and only good will come of forming this connection.

SUMMARY OF THE SEVENTH KEY

- Every disease and every individual are a couple with their own specific path to recovery. No one path and no one solution fits all people.
- Diseases break out in each of us for different reasons, and something different will trigger the internal healing mechanism for every one of us.
- The four primary channels of therapy are as follows:
  - The physiological channel, or how we treat ourselves

(such as eating junk food or hating ourselves). This is the basis for the formation of diseases.

- o The emotional-mental channel, or understanding that the way forward is through the past. Here we seek the emotional source of the disease.
- o The energetic channel, which reminds us that everything in the universe is energy. Our body flows with life energy, and it is possible to cure the body with this energy.
- o The spiritual channel, where a disease occurs when there is no connection between the spirit and matter, between the temporal (everyday self) to the eternal (supernal self).

- Self-awareness leads to wakefulness, where you ask questions and receive answers. Aim your antenna and pick up the broadcast.

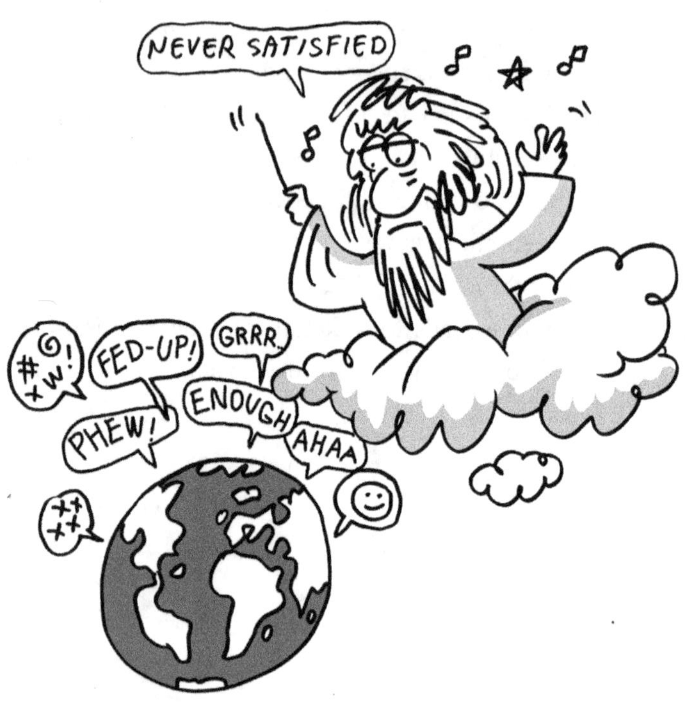

The divine concert prioritizes our supernal good over our immediate good. This can be frustrating and irritating.

FAITH IN THE DIVINE CONCERT

"Research and knowledge lead to faith."

— Anonymous

Let's put the whole issue of God on the table. I am not a religious person, and I probably won't be in this lifetime, since the God I discovered at age forty, after twenty years of faithful atheism, is a God of love and not of retribution, a God of infinite giving and not of fear, a God who appreciates you doing your best, not a God who punishes you for not doing well enough, a God of direct communication, and not a God who requires mediators. The religious institutions and I have different opinions on the subject, and that's fine—we agree to disagree.

I was the greatest of all skeptics. My life circumstances made me one. The first individual who led me to dare think a little differently was Albert Einstein. His many accomplishments impressed me, and I wondered how he reached the conclusion that **coincidences are God's way of remaining anonymous, and that nothing is random, that everything is precise.** When I studied the matter deeply, I came to the conclusion that he was not the only one, and that many other scientists from all over the world had reached the same conclusion: There is a God, there is intelligence behind our creation, the creation of all the universe, and the creation of everything.

I continued to study and began to gather facts that would assist me, a nonscientist, to understand what they had understood that I had missed. We **all agree that design of things is an indication of intelligence**. We are constantly surrounded by man-made products: vehicles, computers, the internet, advanced technologies, art, architecture, and so forth.

None of us ever thinks that they are the result of chance and coincidence. It is obvious to us that a great deal of preliminary design, trial and error, design flaws, and repeated attempts were made until the final product was produced. It is clear to us that metal does not transform itself into a vehicle. It is also clear to us that bolts and springs do not transform themselves into a clock. It is obvious that threads do not weave themselves into a fashionable outfit. It would seem ridiculous to imagine that colored pastes suddenly smeared themselves on a canvas to become the Mona Lisa all on their own. It is likewise obvious that an electrical current does not transform itself into a light bulb, and that processors, chips, and wires do not build themselves into a computer.

So why don't we apply these same assumptions to things that are a thousand times more complicated and complex, such as animals, the human body, everything that grows, or everything hanging up there in the infinite universe? Our mind is incomprehensibly more complicated than the most sophisticated computer that humanity will ever build. Is it not reasonable to assume that if so much planning is required to build a computer, a thousand times as much planning is required to design or create our brains?

An intelligence that creates complexity such as the DNA replication mechanism must be, in and of itself, at least as complex as its own creation, must it not? Likewise for the creation of the universe, whose infinite reaches we cannot even comprehend. What does infinity even mean?

What about our evolution? How we were created? **An evolution based on a process of natural selection is like solving problems without any intelligence or guidance.** It seems to make a lot of sense that no problem is solved without thinking about it, right? There is no comparing an action carried out of intelligence to an action carried out of natural selection, regardless of what those activities are.

It will be all right. **Everything that lives and exists on this planet practically screams intelligent designs. Everything is a testimony to perfection of the divine. Too sublime and high-quality, no way is this chance design. Everything we have created artificially is nothing in comparison to the creation of life itself.**

To this very day, no scientist, no matter what cutting edge technology or sophisticated knowledge employed, has ever been able to create a single living cell, no matter how primitive, and not for lack of trying. Existing cells have been replicated, just as a copier machine does, but have created nothing on their own.

There must be a source that creates life. **Chemical substances do not become living beings on their own. There is no known law of nature, process, or sequence of events that can make new life emerge from inert matter.** So why do we find it so surprising that life is the product of meticulous design? What makes more sense to you? That inert matter transformed into living flesh by chance? The scientific findings indicate a different story.

SYNCHRONICITY, PRECISION, AND PERFECTION

We have come to the divine concert part. Why a concert? Because for a concert to succeed, so that we in the audience can lie back and enjoy the symphony, precision, harmony, and the cooperation of dozens of various musicians, each of which must have their own defined roles—defined instruments, defined sounds, defined locations, even perfectly defined timing. Only cooperation between all of them creates harmonic unity. They simultaneously contribute their outmost, and the sum total is perfect for them all. **Life is like a concert, and God is the conductor. It is all painfully precise, and it all happens at once.**

It is easy for us to appreciate this when good things happen to us, when we are in a good place in our lives, when we get what we want, because it makes us feel that even though the going gets rough occasionally, this moment of perfect harmony makes it all worth it. But when we are in a bad place, we feel the exact opposite. We are angry or sad or feel despair about life, and we don't feel like giving or sharing, and perhaps even hate this terrible life.

Trying to understand how everything occurs simultaneously in this divine concert is like trying to understand how seven billion people could simultaneously search Google, and each of those seven billion people could simultaneously receive, within a fragment of a second, hundreds of thousands of search results. It is inconceivable when you think about it, isn't it? Do any of us (those among us who never studied computer programming) understand how the algorithm residing at the base of this program operates? We are speaking here of a human invention, and we already understood that the one who created the mind of whoever created Google, that same one who created all the great powers in the universe, must be a little more sophisticated, and must possess a few more capabilities than that of this talented inventor.

So perhaps we cannot comprehend with our minds just how everything happens simultaneously or how everything in our lives are precise, but we can still take a few steps to advance us toward accepting the concert and its study that will eventually lead to internalizing the precision of life, so that it will be easier to accept and face the hard and challenging parts in it.

BY CHANCE?

A first lesson in studying the divine concert deals with **reflection about what happened to us in life prior to the current moment, while emphasizing all coincidences that occurred during key points in our lives.** The first thing is to notice everything that happened to you that is defined by the term "by chance." For example, I met such and such a person at such and such a place and at such and such time and heard him say such and such by chance. I chanced to be walking down a different path than usual and saw such and such. I chanced to meet such and such on the bus, I just happened to hear such and such an issue being discussed on the radio. I chanced to quit smoking on that day. I chanced to think of him and just saw him on the street. By chance, by chance, by chance.

In addition, you must note the occurrence of events at key points of your life: selecting a profession, meeting your partner, taking a long vacation abroad, getting laid off, experiencing a divorce, having a wedding. What led to what? Where did you follow your intuition? What did you do that contradicted whatever you believed in so the best or most terrible thing took place?

When you sit down seriously with the words you have written, you can identify how the threads joined and interwove together in order to create, change, and lead you to the next big thing. You can see that in many cases, the question "What are the odds that...?" Leads to the answer "almost none," yet it still happened, in spite of the low odds.

The second lesson in the divine concert is about observation. Start looking at your life in the present, to everything that happens to you, from the moment you wake up in the morning to the moment you pass out in bed. Notice the coincidences that occur and also note the various "I just happened to see" or "I chanced to hear" or "By chance, someone passed by" that others tell you about themselves.

Some will call these observations self-awareness, since you are watching yourself and analyzing what is happening to you and to those around you in real time. **It is true, there is quite a bit of self-awareness in this observation.** Nonetheless, there is also considerable attention to the synchronicity of life, the connection between things, to how everything is linked to everything else, to the thrill that runs through you at events that occurred in spite of the low likelihood of them occurring. It is usually for your greater good and generally leads you to a better place, even if it is different than what you are used to.

The third lesson for the study of the divine concert deals with planning the future and declaring your intentions: What do I want to happen? Most people don't even know what they want, because they don't dare to think about it, because they don't think they deserve to want it, or because they do not have time or sufficient self-awareness to stop and ask themselves this simple question: What do I want? Sit down, investigate, think deeply—seek and you shall find.

The **death exercise** is meant to help you find the things you want to do, realize, or experience in your life. Answer the following questions.

- If the doctor told me today that I would die tomorrow, what would I choose to do?
- If the doctor told me today that I would die in another week, what would I choose to do?
- If the doctor told me today that I would die in another month, what would I choose to do?
- If the doctor told me today that I would die in another year, what would I choose to do?

Answer these questions with all seriousness, as if you have really been told these things. What would you want to accomplish and experience in each of the various timeframes? What would make you happiest? What would make you feel satisfied? What would relieve your heart and mind?

Imagine that you have a year to live and you have to work in that year in order to feed yourself or your family. Would you continue to do what you are doing now? (Most people would not.) Or would you rather choose to do something you always wanted to do as a child but never managed because life happened to you along the way? Be assured that you can learn a great deal about yourself through these questions, through openness to yourself, honesty, and attentiveness to your inner voice.

Once you understand what you want, it is time to consciously choose what you want to accomplish in your life and decide what you are prepared to do to make it happen. Once you understand how all the special things happened to you in the past and how everything is related to everything in the present, you need to understand with both your head and your heart that there is no reason in the world that what you want to happen will happen, that life is precise, and that if something you want is delayed, there must be a reason for it. After all, all other things are precise, and so there is no reason that this specific desire will be exceptional.

It Is All for Our Supernal Good.

There are things that we might want but do not receive. Why don't they happen? Because our own supernal good requires us to be somewhere else, be in some other time, or be with someone else in order to learn, evolve, and grow the most from it. The divine symphony prioritizes our supernal good over our immediate good.

This can be frustrating and irritating because, for the most part, we want things to happen as rapidly as possible, here and now, even if they aren't right for us. The important thing is to have something in your hand. You might really want a specific job, but would be much better off in a different position, whose job interview will not occur for two weeks, because the work environment there is much better suited for you and your needs. You really want the man or woman from last night's date to call you, but they don't really suit you and will only make you miserable. You really want to live abroad right now, but it might be better for you to resolve your ongoing dispute with your parents before you move to another country.

It is hard to understand rationally how the divine concert works, but we can see that it does work by **identifying synchronicity when it happens to us, understanding that it exists, and inducing from it a faith that, at its base, is the supernal good of each one of us.**

This is where we can put the pieces together and link faith in the divine concert to our diseases and our recovery. We are small creators who create reality with our minds, our beliefs, our words, our reactions, and our actions. **The key to health and happiness is to love our creations! To love what we create (even if we created a disease or pain), understanding that that is precisely what we need (even if it hurts), even if it is inconvenient and irritating, and even if we do not understand at that moment why exactly we created what we created.** From then on, we will perform the most precise work for ourselves that can lead us to health and self-realization in all fields of life.

A difficult illness forces us to focus on what is truly important. **A difficult illness forces us to listen to ourselves, to all of our parts, even if it does so in a way that we conceive of at first as being cruel. On the spiritual level, a disease is a tool that we have created out of self-love,** even if on the physical and emotional level it is self-hatred that generated the disease.

It is love of our true essence, of our potential, of our ability to realize ourselves in the highest level. **It is a love that forces us to change, that forces us to want to change, and it requires a great deal of patience for ourselves and the process.** Things do not happen when we want, but instead when it is most right for them to happen, if it is right for them to happen at all. We assume responsibility with the inner knowledge and understanding that if all good and all bad things that have occurred to us in the past have led to our emotional, mental, and spiritual growth, evolution, and education, there is no reason for this trend to reverse itself now that we have chosen to assume responsibility for our creation, for the disease, and for healing ourselves.

All we need to do is be thankful for what we have received and all that we have, and to be attentive to ourselves, to all of our parts. I will conclude this chapter with the words of Dr. Deepak Chopra: **"Our brain is programmed to know God."** We are programmed to find Him. The program is installed on our hard disks. Even if He has chosen to be invisible, even if we never hear His voice, our heart will feel Him because emotion is the bridge connecting the day-to-day and the supernal worlds.

SUMMARY OF THE EIGHTH KEY

- Planning things requires wisdom. It is not a function of time and coincidence.
- We live within a divine concert in which everything is synchronized with everything else, and nothing, nothing at all, is random. The emphasis of this symphony is our supernal good and not our immediate good.
- Look backward in life to what has happened and note all of the coincidences that have occurred, particularly at key points in your life.
- Look upon your life in the present and seek synchronicity.
- Understand what your desires are and select what you choose to achieve in your life.
- A severe illness pushes us to listen to ourselves, to all of our parts, even if the road to this seems cruel at first.
- On the spiritual level, disease is a tool we create out of self-love that forces us to change.

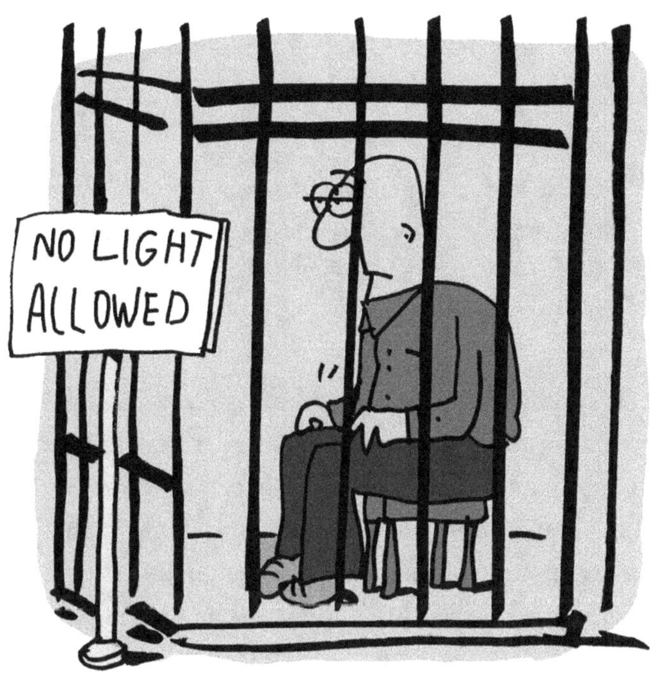

If concepts like "the light," unity, God, souls, angels, reincarnation, aliens, auras, spiritual entities, or karma give you the chills, nausea, or any other kind of reflexive repugnant reaction, skip to the next chapter.

NOT FOR THE FAINT OF HEART

> *"We can easily forgive a child who is afraid of the dark; the real tragedy of life is when men are afraid of the light."*
>
> — Plato

This chapter is not intended for those who believe that their life is just fine the way it is.[6] There is a certain danger in reading materials that can shatter or change everything you think you know about life and the prism through which you have chosen to observe and respond to life. It requires a good helping of courage to be open to a change that might be life-changing without immediately rejecting it. After all, this change does not fit any pattern or formula you are familiar with.

It is important to note that you need not read this chapter in order to get well. Everything written up to this point is more than enough for most of you. If words like

---

6   This chapter was inspired by material I was exposed to in the Migdalor (Lighthouse) Center by Ilana Rogel, author of the encyclopedia *Of Spirit and Matter*.

light, spiritual unity, divinity, souls, angels, reincarnation, aliens, auras, entities, or karma give you chills, nausea, or any other kind of adverse reaction, skip to the final chapter.

The questions of existence before and after life as a human being, existence before birth, and existence after death have always preoccupied mankind, and for good reason.

"What—you are born, you live, you die, and that's it? Food, sex, laughs, children, and a few slaps on the face along the way and it's all over?"

"Are we alone in the universe or is there life on other planets?"

"What really happens to all those who die, see a tunnel of light, and then come back to tell the tale?"

"What is all this business about miracles?"

"Are there ghosts or aren't there?"

There are plenty of questions with no clear-cut answers. I make no pretensions of unlocking here the secrets of life and creation, or revealing the secret thoughts of God when He saw fit to create an orb rotating in the void around a massive sphere of flaming gas. What I will do is condense what I have learned, read, and studied, both externally and internally over the past decade regarding the creator, creation, and our purpose in life. I'll try to do this while using the simplest language possible and, of course, tie it in to the subjects of health and illness. That is why you are reading this book, after all, isn't it?

Let's start with an axiomatic statement (a self-evident assumption that requires no proof): **We exist before and**

after death. Those are the findings of my research in which I was exposed to thousands of stories from people all over the world who have experienced a taste of that divine place. This included hundreds of scientific studies that investigated the issue over 150 years ago (a wonderful book that condenses several dozen of them is *Life After Death* by D. Scott Rogo), thousands of channeling sessions from hundreds of sentient, non-corporeal entities that transmit information to us, hundreds of confirmed testimonies of children who recalled every detail of their previous incarnations, and ancient and wise cultures from all over the world who spoke of it.

I ended up returning to my own cultural roots through the Old Testament, which contains within it the codes of the universe, and the Kabbalah, which cracks those codes. They both tell the same basic story as the holy books of other religions, once you get past culture-specific idiosyncrasies. As far as I was concerned, it was the only rational conclusion I could accept. The same story repeated itself in thousands of versions throughout thousands of years of human history. I would have been crazy if I had continued to ignore this juxtaposition.

So why are we actually here?

The source of creation—the divinity, the infinite divine energy that created and creates all in existence—has decided to experience itself through manifestation in the flesh. A portion of it split off and scattered into billions of shards. Those shards reach the flesh and spirit laboratory called Earth for an experiential, educational journey. **The divine watches "them" (its extensions) without judging**

or interfering in their journey, as it experiences and manifests itself. These fragments are those through which the divine senses the world.

Each shard, each spark of God, is an energetic and eternal entity (a meaningful and existent essence). A very small part of that essence enters into this world as a condensed and limited physical body (yes, that's each and every one of us), having agreed **to play a memory game on this Earth. This game requires it (us) to deliberately forget the place it came from, the reason it came here, and the incredible essence that it is** in order to do the following:

- Learn about itself through emotional experiences
- Make restitution for the errors of past incarnations and grow beyond them
- (Changes and modifications to the spirit can only be carried out through the mediation of matter.)
- Fulfill and realize its task and role, the primordial-spiritual contract that it has signed

Do you now understand why so many sources define God as living within us as the progeny of God? It is because we contain within ourselves minute fragments of the divine, and they instill the spirit of life within us.

Every spirit, prior to its arrival on Earth, carefully plots out that specific pulse of life, that specific incarnation. Each and every parameter is carefully examined in accordance with the spiritual contract and in accordance to its history on previous incarnations, whether on Earth or on other planets.

Yes, even civilizations living in other galaxies have spirits. We call them aliens, and they likely call us "that arrogant species that has yet to understand what kind of universe they live in, but already thinks they know everything." The game their spirits play is the same as that of our own, with one small difference: **Here on Earth, the gap between the higher frequencies in which the light entity vibrates to the lower frequency in which the condensed physical body vibrates is the greatest in the entire cosmos.**

This laboratory is a focus of interest for the entire cosmos due to this incredibly wide gap, which is unique to human beings. **The research questions examined on this planet are: Can one reach the supernal heights from a starting point that is so low? Can we, from a victimized, polar, despairing place lacking in self-worth, recall our eternal and magnificent essence and reach self-realization, happiness, and unconditional love? Can we, out of separation, select unity?**

Our planet might be the most difficult, but it is also the most educational and the most experiential. At the end of the day, the only thing we take from here is the collection of emotional experiences, and there are quite a few of those to be had in this world.

EVERY ONE OF US IS UNIQUE AND SPECIAL

Each and every spirit is unique and special and has its own essence, character, role, and characteristics, just like every one of us has a unique fingerprint. **Each spirit carefully selects, in accordance with its own particular lessons and what it wishes to learn and experience, the following: its gender, nationality, skin color, residential area, family members, friends, and opportunities; life buoys scattered along the path it has chosen; different exit points according to progress or realization; and what it wishes to face, how, and with whom, including the blows it will suffer that will enable it to experience certain experiences.**

It does not plan it on its own, but does so together with its guides, highly evolved and experienced entities of light, and with spirits clustered with it who share the same level of spiritual evolution and who reincarnate in synchronization with it. On Earth, these spirits attract each other so that they can help each other realize the various clauses of the contract they have signed.

Most of us do not have a sterling performance record here on Earth, to put it mildly. In fact, some of us murder, steal, harm, rape, fight, corrupt, or bully and prey on those weaker than us, and have done so since the dawn of humanity. Accordingly, when the eternal essence leaves the temporal body-soul, physical-mental vessel—when it returns to the source and examines, together with its guides, the significant events in its life (and they are all significant)—reand its often poor performance in the trials it has undergone—it feels incredible distress, since the source it has come from is a place of infinite love and compassion, whereas the actions it performed under the veil of forgetfulness are terrible by any measure.

It will have to repeat the lessons it has failed, because you cannot graduate to second grade before finishing the first. One of the reasons the spirit finds it so difficult to ascend is **the eternal conflict between the desires and passions of the temporal body-soul to the desires of the eternal spirit.** In an ideal world, the spirit is the planning authority—the mastermind, the one that desires, dreams, and yearns—and the soul-body is the executing authority that carries out the desires of the spirit. The spirit communicates its desires to the physical body through emotion, and it hopes that it will make its dreams reality.

In other words, life is not really just a dialogue between the body and the soul, but a three-way conversation in which the spirit, soul, and body participate. The spirit transmits its desires through emotion, indicating whether it does or does not approve of the action undertaken by the body, the situation being experienced, a word or person it is exposed to, and whether this is right or wrong for it.

That is how the spirit creates matter. The body-soul does not always feel like moving in the direction the spirit attempts to indicate. It wants to go left but they feel like going right; it wants action, but they want quiet. **There is a consistent and unending conflict between the temporal and eternal parts that make up a human being.**

The Soul As a Reflection of the Spirit

Now let's connect this to the issue of disease and health. **A disease is the language of the soul, and the soul is a reflection of the spirit.** When the spirit selects the body-soul into which it enters, it selects a soul whose emotional and perceptive components are identical to its own.

For example, if the spirit wishes to investigate self-worth, it will choose a soul with low self-worth. If the spirit wishes to experience and investigate self-victimization, it will choose a soul whose biography has made it a victim. If the spirit wishes to experience evil so that it might learn about good, it will select a soul whose life will lead it to commit evil deeds. If the spirit wishes to practice sexual self-control, it will select a soul that is fated to become a sex addict.

The soul is a reflection of the spirit and the goals it seeks to accomplish. If, in the framework of the struggle for control between the body-soul and the spirit, the former are victorious—for example by life flowing in the direction they seek (such as working in Wall Street instead of writing self-improvement books, though the opposite could be equally true)—the spirit despairs, gives up hope, and is shunted aside, and that is when all the chronic and autoimmune diseases show up.

Man has turned against himself, against his spirit, against his true desires. **No reality has been created here that has not been taken into consideration as an option prior to the arrival on this planet. Disease is an option that the spirit has taken with it on this specific journey, and it**

can either be realized or not. No one can create anything that did not potentially exist as an option to begin with.

The verse "All is foreseen, but freedom of choice is given"[7] can be understood in this context. All the possible choices and possible paths are known in advance. What remains unknown is which free choice will actually be exercised and which path the soul seeks to follow.

An individual who wishes to heal himself—who wishes to assume responsibility for his creation, for his disease, even if it was formed subconsciously—must work toward achieving unity between the two parts within him, to minimize the conflict as much as possible. We can do that by creating proper conditions to listen and being attentive to this inner voice, the voice of the spirit, the supernal part of us.

This is not a one-time event. This is a path that must be walked consistently, until this pulse of life is completed. The answers and the unity between the opposing desires does not come at once, and full unity might never be achieved, due to the fundamental difference between the two factors. However, it is certainly possible to reach a fertile collaboration between the two.

This involves training, which takes time. But the first step is the most important one: the awakening and recollection of your eternal essence. Afterward will come the desire

---

7   By Rabbi Akiva, a Jewish wise man who lived in the second-century Christian era and is considered to be one of the great luminaries of Judaism.

to attach yourself to it and act together toward the realization of your supernal vision. **In this way, you will be able to transition from internal doubt to internal satisfaction. From "I am not sufficiently loved, not sufficiently appreciated, and not sufficiently worthy" to "I am loved. I am appreciated. I am worthy."**

You will never have proof of the existence of this spirit. You will never be able to place the spirit, or God, under a microscope. You will never be able to see or touch them. Even if you could, what would be the point? What would be the challenge? What would be the quest? What would be the free choice between assertion and negation? Between good and evil? Between unity and separation? What would be the journey made, the wisdom gained, or the lesson learned? Accordingly, the only thing we can do is feel them in our hearts. That is our only option.

SUMMARY OF THE CHAPTER

- We are the fingers through which the divine feels and experiences the world.
- The spirit forgets its origins in order to learn, fix itself, and realize the spiritual contract.
- The spirit is the planning authority, the mastermind that desires, dreams, and seeks out, and the body is the executive authority carrying out these desires.
- The spirit communicates its desires to the material body through emotion.

- Disease is an option for realization that the spirit has taken you with it on this specific journey. Nothing can be created that was not an option all along.
- A man who desires to cure himself must act to achieve unity between the two parts within him, the eternal and the temporal.

PART 3

THE PERSONAL JOURNEY OF HEALING

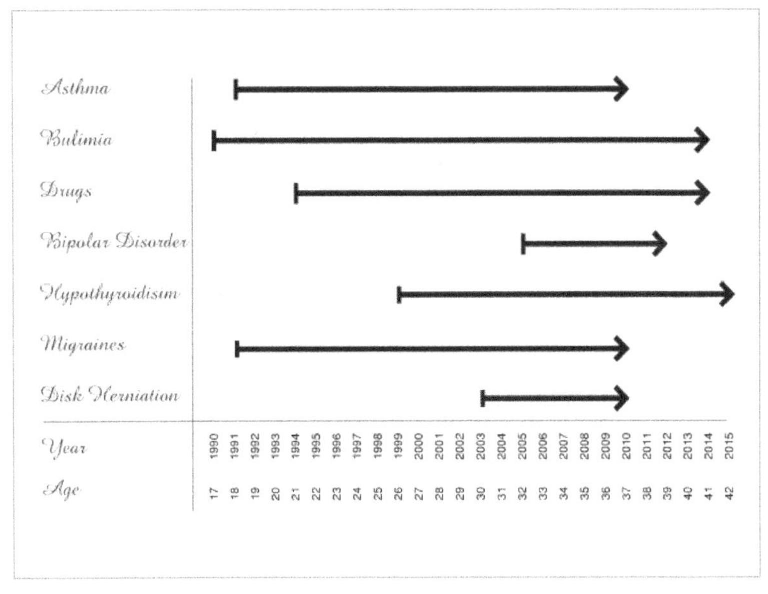

CHAPTER 1
THE FIRST STEP

It isn't that I got up one fine morning and said, "Hell with it. I'm sick and tired of being dependent on pills, so I'm going to read up on how to free myself from them." Nothing could be further from the truth.

Furthermore, I never viewed myself as being "ill." I always viewed myself as being a very healthy woman who just happens to suffer from a few unrelated diseases. Even though the list of permanent diagnostic conditions in my HMO sheet was as long as a nineteenth-century Russian novel, when asked if I was generally healthy, I usually answered, "Of course!"

And it isn't that I was being deceptive or dishonest, or that I felt I was being self-deceptive or in denial. I honestly believed that I was a healthy person, mentally as well as physically. Even when the psychiatrist pronounced me to be manic-depressive, an inner voice told me that I was fine, that I was healthy, that there wasn't really anything wrong with my head. I didn't really believe the psychiatrist, but I still devoured the pills he offered me, because I didn't want to be depressed anymore.

So what spurred me to leave the semi-denial niche I had occupied since I was seventeen and a half, when all of my myriad medical conditions began to appear until I was thirty-six, when I decided to cure myself of asthma? It was an echo of a sentence uttered by a friend with whom I shared my diagnosis of hypothyroidism, which meant that my thyroid gland was not producing the hormones my body required and that for the rest of my life, I would have to take pills containing the hormone that the deficient gland was not supplying.

At the time, I was thirty-three, and my good friend said nonchalantly, "Welcome to the thirties' pills," then explained to me that in the United States (where he had spent his youth following relocation required by the company where his father was employed), it was a common term, since everyone in their thirties started taking pills of some sort or another to balance out one deficient bodily function or another, regardless of their overall health. He compared the casual acceptance of the thirties-onward pill regimen in the U.S. to Israelis casual acceptance of mandatory military service at age eighteen and reserve duty thereafter. Just one of those life stages that seems odd from the outside but completely normal from the inside.

This sentence resonated with me for a long time and troubled me deeply. Something within me rejected the fact that I, only in my thirties, suddenly found myself dependent on so many pills. It made me feel old and decrepit.

So I made a list of all the pills I took on a daily basis. It was a long list.

- Steroids and Ventolin inhalers for asthma
- Antidepressants for my depression
- Powerful painkillers to deal with both my migraines and a nasty disc herniation
- And the latest acquisition, Eltroxin, to counter my hypothyroidism

In addition to this chemical cocktail, I kept my bulimia carefully hidden from the entire world. I also smoked light drugs on a daily basis, which really did make my life seem more tolerable. Such was my life in those days, and that is why that sentence "Welcome to your thirties' pills" did not fail to resonate.

One day, I saw a movie about cancer patients in their terminal stage who had all been informed they were going to die, quite literally. Conventional medicine had given up on them and advised them to say their farewells to their families and loved ones and wait for death to come.

They underwent a particularly radical treatment that included various organic vegetable juices and enemas, something which I then viewed as delusional. And yet, all of the people interviewed for the movie did so ten to twenty years after being sent to die—and they all seemed healthy and happy.

Aristotle, the father of scientific inquiry, said thousands of years ago that the inception of science is wonderment, and that was what I felt when I saw people condemned to death so many years ago who were still alive. How could it be that something like this was even possible, and that I had never heard about it before?

That was the first step of my journey toward healing. I had not yet embarked on the journey, and I had not yet declared that I was going to cure myself and be healthy, because I did not yet believe that it was truly possible. I simply started reading, watching, and slowly enabling myself to change the belief system that had led me to the sick place where I found myself without hope or faith that something could change.

I will try to summarize those essentials of my self-education during the first four difficult years, which touched me most deeply, so that we might progress to the actual journey toward self-curing.

The body is a massive masterwork machine that always strives toward eternal balance and is programmed accordingly. People like you and I will never know just how smart, sophisticated, and complex this system is. Trillions of parts interacting with trillions of other parts every second and every minute of the day, 24/7, with no break for holidays. These trillions of interactions occur near simultaneously with divine synchronization and with no intervention on our part. This magical system has an innate ability to heal. It is built-in—that is how it arrives from God's factory.

It doesn't matter what horrors you inflict on this system—slice it up, burn it, shatter it, infect it with viruses or bacteria, or poison it—regardless, the system knows how to return to equilibrium. It really doesn't need any help from anyone. Our immune system knows what it needs to do in order to eliminate external invaders or make whole a bone fracture or wound or burn. That's just how nature is designed.

But what about autoimmune diseases that, once diagnosed, are never cured and turn us into pill-dependent junkies for life? Suddenly, the body attacks itself. That very same high-performance immune system, as mighty and super-smart as it is, suddenly grows confused, identifies components of the body as foreign invaders, and destroys them. The machine goes "bonkers," to put it in simple terms.

But the analogy is flawed. Machines designed by humans can break down and malfunction, but the machines designed by nature (the universe, the creator, the source, or God, the primordial energy) do not malfunction. If there is a problem, the system is programmed to deal with it and restore itself to balance and equilibrium at all costs. So why does the system turn against itself all of a sudden? Does it have suicidal tendencies? What the hell is going on here?

Doctors have all this information. They have, after all, spent many years studying this machine. They simply never stop to ask *why* John Doe's machine lost its equilibrium. Why are the masterwork gears creaking all of a sudden? Why has the brilliant design lost its luster?

When I asked my endocrinologist why my body was attacking my thyroid gland, the answer I got was that was just the way it is. Autoimmune diseases just break out and nobody knows why. My doctor said, "So just accept it, take your pills, and move on, because there is nothing else you can do."

Let me use another specific example that many self-healing books use that is very simple to understand and demonstrates a general and very important principal. Say you are driving your car and the fuel warning light switches on. What would you do? Drive into a gas station, of course. Now suppose that the gas station attendant shows up and tells you, "I will handle your problem." Then you see him switch off your fuel warning light, smile, and tell you, "That's it. Problem solved. Godspeed!"

What would you say? Probably something like "Are you serious? Why did you switch off the warning light? The fuel warning light is fine, it's operating just like it's supposed to. The car needs gas!" Right? Then understand that if something is wrong with your digestive tract—and it doesn't really matter whether the problem is diarrhea, constipation, heartburn, or cramps—that problem is the warning light indicating that you are out of gas. That is how your body is signaling you. "Hello, buddy! Something here is wrong. Something here is out of equilibrium. Please pay attention to it."

When you choose to solve the problem by taking a pill, you are simply shutting off the lamp without addressing the real problem, the root cause that caused the light to appear in the first place. You are temporarily suppressing the symptom, but not curing the source of the problem. Eventually, your vehicle will grind to a halt because you did not deal with the source of the problem. You did not gas up; instead, you just switched off the warning light informing you that you were about to run out of gas.

What is the root source of our body's warning light? We

need to dig in and consider possible causes on a case-by-case basis; there are no ready-made answers. It may be that it is physical, it may be that it is mental-emotional, or it may be both. Simple to understand, right?

So why do we find it so ridiculously easy to understand the empty gas tank analogy, but so hard to understand and accept that is also exactly what is happening with our bodies? Why do we rush off to take a pill and switch off the warning light imploring us to deal with the problem every time we have some sort of pain? This is what we do, again and again, throughout our lives. The deep understanding of this repetitive behavior and its mechanism was essential for me and for my healing journey.

Looking backward, what most touched me and spurred me on my path of self-healing, far more than everything I learned about the human body and self-healing techniques, were the thousands of personal testimonies of people who had succeeded against all odds and in total contradiction to their doctors' prognoses to recover from terminal or incurable illnesses. People who dared to live, to disregard and defy the fate pronounced for them by the medical system.

I noticed two things in particular. The first is that they all believed it was possible. An inner voice told them not to give up. The other thing is that it was easier, paradoxically, for those people who were condemned to death, whom conventional medicine had given up on, to begin the journey than for people who suffered from non-terminal or life-threatening illnesses.

This makes a lot of sense if you stop to think about it; they had nothing to lose. The angel of death was knocking at the door, and all conventional medicine had to tell them was to let him in! It was exactly this stance that impelled them to find their own answers and own paths to health. They were prepared to listen, to make changes, to make an effort, regardless of how the answers sounded or the responses they received from their environments.

CHAPTER 2
ASTHMA

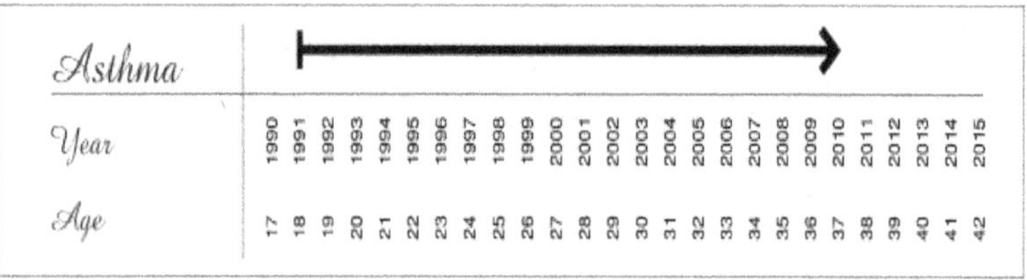

The first disease I overcame was asthma. One day, I just got up and decided that enough was enough! I was tired of my constant asthma attacks, I was tired of the inhalers, and I was tired of steroids. I had just had enough of being asthmatic, enough of being ill.

My asthma had started without any early warning at age eighteen, just after I joined the army. Until then, I had been a healthy girl who was never ill, but that first asthma attack led to my first week-long hospitalization. My most salient memory of this time, beyond being the only hospitalized individual in the wing under the age of seventy, was that the doctors kept grilling me about whether I was quite sure that I had never suffered an asthma seizure in the past. I remember wondering whether they thought that the answer would change between one visit to the doctor to the next.

Eighteen years, dozens of hospitalizations, thousands of steroid pills, and hundreds of inhalers later, I said, "Enough! This far and no further. If terminal patients have been able to save themselves from certain death and recover, there is no reason that I cannot cure myself of this asthma." At that time, I was already suffering from an active bipolar disorder, which I was concealing from everyone, just like I was concealing my bulimia. In addition, I was suffering from constant back pains, migraines, and hypothyroidism.

So, what do we do? Who do we turn to? How do we begin? I had a great deal of scattered information in my head, some inspiration from others, and absolutely no action plan. To be completely honest, I didn't really believe I could completely cure my asthma, because my family doctor had laughed in my face and even mocked me when I shared my cunning scheme to get well. He told me I was wasting my time and efforts and setting myself up for disappointment, because "with lungs like yours, this won't happen. I've been treating you for enough years to be sure of that."

I decided that I would prove him wrong. I would show him what's what. This contrariness gave me the kick in the rear end that I needed to undertake the actual journey and take action. That kick constituted the termination of my preparatory maturation period.

During this period, which lasted several years, I acquired knowledge, increased my self-confidence, and developed immunity to the mockery that was my lot every time I shared my intentions to get well and cure my diseases with my friends and relatives. It isn't that they didn't want me to be well, they just didn't believe it was possible, just like my doctor didn't believe it was possible. Some of them were afraid that I was going to do myself harm, and some of them thought that I was going through some kind of mental breakdown. Those who were most concerned shared their concerns with my husband and even recommended that we think about some sort of appropriate psychological treatment.

I didn't really believe I could make it, but I did believe that something had to change. My journey to self-healing proceeded in four channels: mental, energetic, physical, and spiritual.

THE FIRST CHANNEL: THE CHANNEL OF THE SOUL

At that point in time, I was treated by a psychiatrist for about four years after my first depression. Four years earlier, my psychiatrist had sent me to a psychologist, saying that the pills he prescribed would only balance my brain chemistry, but that I also had to treat my soul.

He was right. I spent a month and a half with her. She helped me a great deal and was very nice. There was only one problem: I have no idea what we talked about. I was not really ready to start sharing what was really troubling me. How do I know that? Because I never told her that my father had beaten me throughout my childhood. I kept that minor matter secret from her. I didn't dare utter the phrase "my father beat me."

Part of me was still ashamed of being a battered child, and besides, as far as I was concerned, he had died so many years ago. (My father passed away from cancer when I was twenty years old.) So why bother opening up that can of worms? He was dead and not coming back, so there was no one to blame and no one to shout at. So thanks but no thanks. I will let sleeping dogs lie.

Toward the end of that treatment, my pills began to take effect. I felt wonderful, and my smile and zest for life had seemingly returned. The psychologist and I said farewell as friends.

Four years later, I was in a different mental and emotional place. I wanted to cure myself from a chronic disease and knew that body, mind, and soul were one, which meant that diseases were interlinked and derived to some extent from our soul. It felt right to go to back to psychological therapy. The right time had come, and I felt ready to share with my new therapist the fact that my father had beaten me throughout my entire childhood, in spite of me being a well-behaved daughter and student who earned top grades.

I had never understood why I deserved this treatment and why my father could transform in a second into such a monster. I also shared with her another secret: For many years, I wished my father would die. Every time he beat me for no good reason, I would stare up at the sky and cry out, "Please, let him die. Please, please make him die. I can't live with him anymore."

So when he eventually did get cancer and die, I felt guilty, which is part of what we talked about—my repressed guilt and feelings that I had killed my father. We talked about my sense of humiliation and injustice at being beaten all those years, about my love-hate relationship with him, and how hard it was to contain the conflicts in the narrative of "I love my father. We had good times and special moments together. We both had dreams of me becoming a doctor one day. I miss him so much," and "Why did he do this to me? How could he? Why did I deserve it? I hope he rots in Hell."

I started weeping nonstop in my meetings with her. Understand, for many years I had not wept at all. I was emotionally sealed off. My feelings were all barricaded behind reinforced concrete walls. That was how I protected myself after years of insults and humiliation. In my sessions with her, I felt that rivers of grief and anger were flowing out of me for the first time in many years, making some space for something new. My soul began to feel lighter.

Aside from this emotional catharsis, the therapist granted me, for the first time in my life, a psychological understanding of the **timing** of my diseases. Both the asthma and the migraines began immediately after I left home and joined the army. She explained to me that by leaving home, I had been rescued from **physical abuse, and seemingly survived the emotional hell I had experienced for so many years as a child and a teenage girl, but my body still remembered this abuse, and my soul neither forgot nor forgave it. This was expressed in the disease that had erupted, all of a sudden and with no early warning.** I remember that in that moment she explained all this to me,

I simply knew that this was the reason. Somehow knowing this answered all of the doubts I had over the years, which I had never been able to resolve on my own.

During that time, two other things also happened. Seemingly, they had nothing to do with each other but, as life has taught me, everything in life is interconnected. One day I met a healer, a friend of a good friend, who invited me to a session at her home. I told her I was undergoing so many different kinds of treatments and therapies at the time that I could not afford anything else, and she told me that she was offering to treat me for free because that is what "they" had asked her to do.

I did not know back then who "they" were, why she would be willing to do as "they" asked, or what she did in her sessions, but I trusted my friend, who told me that the healer had performed literal miracles for those she had treated.

I underwent a few healing sessions with her, and some of those sessions included guided imagery exercises. All I can say about her healing technique is that I lay on a therapeutic bed while she moved around the room and manipulated the energies around me. I didn't feel anything physically, not even prickles or goosebumps on my skin, let alone pressure in my head or elevated heartbeats or any of the other physical symptoms I had read or heard about from other people who had undergone similar experiences. Still, I knew **something** was happening, that this something was taking place on a level I could not intellectually comprehend, and that it was positive and beneficial for me.

In one of my guided imagery sessions, I reached a

situation where I passed through imaginings of myself at several different ages (eight, twelve, sixteen, and eighteen). In these imaginings, my father and I sat next to a fire, and then the healer asked me what I wanted to do to my father.

I responded, "To beat him up, to punish him."

At that moment, all four characters—me at different ages—began beating the shit out of my father. There is simply no other way to describe it. I simply beat him violently, with as much fury and outrage as I could summon—and I could summon quite a bit.

Throughout the imaging, the characters cursed and screamed their pent-up pain, my pent-up pain. It lasted several minutes and I did not stop weeping the entire time. This violent imaging was one of the most powerful things I had ever experienced, and when I was done—partially because I felt drained of strength to continue and partially because I felt that I was ready to move on—all of the characters joined into one, and I hugged my father.

I loved him so much at that moment that suddenly the thought of forgiving him didn't seem so strange. Suddenly, there was no room in me for the "I will never forgive him for what he did to me" narrative.

In my next session with my therapist, I told her about the experience. She was very excited and happy for me and said that this was one of the best outcomes I could have hoped for, because the girls within me had done in their imagination what I had never dared do in real life because of the fear that had paralyzed me, every time anew, every time I was beaten. They had protected themselves and retaliated for their (my) victimization, and thereby released volumes of pent-up hatred, anger, and frustration.

The other development that occurred during that time, also somewhat odd, took place following a session with a medium I contacted, following a recommendation by another friend. As soon as I sat down, she told me, "Your father's energy is here because he wants you to know that he is not at all angry at you, so you shouldn't feel guilty. He is very proud of who you are, what you do, and the family you have raised, and he is always looking out for you."

I didn't understand where she was coming up with this, and I didn't know how to digest or process the message that she had claimed to "pass on" to me from my father. I left her feeling very confused but surprisingly relaxed, and from the moment I entered my car until the moment I parked it by my home, I couldn't stop crying. For nearly thirty minutes, I couldn't stop the flow of the most powerful tears that I had ever wept, even more powerful than my tears during the guided imagery where my younger "selves" had retaliated against my father.

I returned to the medium a few days later, after I'd had a chance to think about her message. I told her that assuming what she told me was true (even though it sounded completely nuts) and my father's "energy," was still in the room with me, I wanted to ask his forgiveness for wishing him dead so many times over so many years. To my surprise, the medium claimed "my father" was no longer there. She said that he had passed on the message that was important for him to pass on and had moved on.

When I told her about the psychological therapy I was undergoing and how much anger I felt toward how he had treated me as a child, she just looked at me and calmly stated, "I don't know what you want from him. On the spiritual level, he did exactly what you asked him to do. That was the contract you two made before either of you arrived in this world, and he kept his end of the bargain. You have no cause for complaint against him. On the contrary, you should thank him. It is only thanks to him that you became who you are today."

I was angry when she said that. No, I was furious. I thought, "What an evil woman. How can she say something like that to me? I lived out my entire childhood in a state of emotional terror, afraid of the next beating." But at the same time, this anger was accompanied by a vague understanding that her words were essentially true. This understanding was not, of course, on the rational-intellectual level, nor did it exist on the emotional level, but I still felt it hovering somewhere in my soul, and so I let it go.

A few days later, in a session with my therapist, I told her that I felt I was prepared to forgive my father. I do not know where my insight came from, but I suddenly comprehended his limitations and flaws, understood his difficulty in dealing with who he was, understood that he had been beaten badly as a child and that this was the only means of education and child-rearing that he had known.

I understood that he could not grow past it the way I had, because when I was beaten I swore to myself that I would never raise a hand to my children, that they would never feel what I was feeling. That, at least, was one vow that I always managed to keep. I understood that he was weaker than I was and that I was the strong one, and I just let it go and forgave him his weaknesses. I returned to feeling love toward him.

The Second Channel: The Energetic Channel

I continued going to the healer, even though I felt no physical sensation during her energetic treatments. It just felt right, and more importantly I somehow felt she knew what she was doing. In parallel, I started undergoing a series of treatments with a chiropractor who worked in collaboration with other alternative medicine practitioners. I defined myself to them as being in the process of self-healing from asthma and that I felt I needed to help my body during the process.

Aside from the chiropractor (who was also an enthusiastic Kabbalist), I also underwent acupuncture, shiatzu, tui na, reflexology, even suction-cup therapy, many of them common treatment techniques in traditional Chinese medicine.

I heard a whole slew of various explanations of the life energy that flows through our bodies in energy channels and about how blockages in those channels can be expressed as pain and diseases. I heard about the importance of pinpointing and treating the source of a disease rather than the symptomatic treatment of its symptoms, and a great deal about the body's innate ability to heal itself.

I didn't always understand why the various alternate

medicine practitioners kept telling me stuff like "Today we will treat the spleen" or "Today we will treat the pancreas," when I had made clear that I was looking for treatment of my lungs. Since I never really understood all of their explanations, I just intuitively assumed that just as I didn't understand many things about what conventional doctors did, I just had to trust they knew what they were doing.

I also always encouraged the alternate medicine practitioners to share with me the success stories of other patients, and this lifted my spirits and strengthened my resolve to stay the course. Throughout, they provided me with a great deal of support and encouragement for the path I had undertaken. My general feeling was that I was in the right place.

Not everything was rosy. I also received nutritional instructions, which I failed to fully carry out. I felt that my nutrition was fine as it was, since I was careful to eat vegetables every day and avoided eating too much junk and sugar products. But to be honest, the main reason I didn't follow their nutritional instructions was that I just didn't feel like ending dairy product consumption. I subsisted on cottage cheese, hard cheeses, and other dairy products, and I just wasn't ready to give them up, even though that was the first instruction I received. I simply hadn't matured enough to accept that nutritional change, which was very radical for me, and even my fierce desire to get well couldn't impel me to follow those instructions.

THE THIRD CHANNEL: THE PHYSICAL CHANNEL

I received from my various therapists a list of breathing exercises to perform at home, and I carried them out faithfully, partially in order to mollify my guilt at refusing to give up dairy products. What was nice about that "homework" is that it inspired me to take initiative. I decided intuitively to do everything I could to expand my respiratory volume. What did that mean in practice? Doing everything to expand the volume of my clogged-up lungs, as I perceived them.

Throughout the day, I would spit out phlegm while repeating the mantra "I am expelling all of the poison from my lungs." I really worked at it, clearing my throat dozens of times each day, creating a lump of phlegm and spitting it out while directing my mind and heart to the mantra.

Another thing I did each day was expand the volume of my lungs by holding my breath and completing imagery work. I would fill my lungs with air, as if I were diving underwater, close my eyes, and imagine how the air was pushing against the sides of my lungs which in turn were stretching and expanding, creating space for more air in the next breath.

Care to guess when I had time to perform this little drill? Well, since I was working full-time plus extra hours, and since I was raising small children, this meant I had almost no free time. So what I did was devote my restroom time to breathing exercises.

THE FINAL CHANNEL: THANKFULNESS

A year or two before I started my self-healing journey, I watched the film *The Secret* with a spiritual friend. In the film, the characters spoke about how like attracts like, and that the way to deal with someone who irritates you was to project positive thoughts at them instead of cursing at them. At the time, I was a columnist and I had an editor who supervised my column and treated me badly, with no justification.

I decided to make her into my lab rat and try out this technique on her. At first this was not simple, to put it mildly, because I was so used to responding to her text messages and emails with "What does this X want from me?" (Fill in X with your favorite profanity. Hint: In my case, it included unsympathetic animals.) Still, I literally forced myself to stand in her shoes, and try to feel what was going on in her mind and leading her to respond to me as she did. After all, there must have been a reason that a young, otherwise fortunate, and successful woman was so angry all day.

I started sending her empowering messages, congratulations, and greetings. Nothing too complicated, just simple stuff like "I wish you the best in life," "May you enjoy a good relationship," "I wish you love from all around you," and all sorts of other such well wishes. And lo and behold, within a few months, her attitude toward me turned around completely. Since we did not have a personal relationship, I do not know what changed in her life during that period, if anything. All I can testify to is her attitude toward me.

Seemingly, neither her previously hostile attitude toward me nor her later improved attitude had any cause. The only thing that changed was my mental attitude toward her.

Let's get back to my journey of self-healing. Aside from the change my editor underwent, the primary impression left in my mind from that movie was the concept of thankfulness, the importance of thanking and praising the universe for all we have and all we try to create. That is why I used every opportunity I had to thank myself for having the strength to cure myself with every wad of phlegm I spat out. It felt right to me to thank not the universe but myself for taking this step, for liberating myself from the illness that had accompanied me throughout my adult life.

After four months, I decided that my efforts had been successful and that I was healthy, so I asked my pulmonologist for a referral to a lung institute, which would perform a fateful examination to determine whether my concentrated efforts, including my crazy, intuitive breathing drills, had worked. The pulmonologist wished me well, but I could see he was skeptical and was just humoring me.

I came back to the pulmonologist two weeks later, a ball of nerves since I did not know what the test results meant. I tried to question the technician who had performed the tests on me, but she refused to share the meaning of the results and dryly answered, "Ma'am, only a doctor can interpret the results. Ask him." The doctor looked at the form, read the results, looked at me, scratched his head, and said, "From what I can see, it looks like you succeeded."

I was unable to process his answer and asked in return,

"But what does that mean?"

He answered, "It means that whatever you did, you probably did it well, because these are the results of an individual with properly functioning lungs."

Still unable to process this achievement, I asked, "That means my family doctor can delete the asthma diagnosis from my online medical record? I can press delete?"

The doctor laughed and answered, "I don't know what you did, but yes, you can press delete."

Every individual has a few defining moments in his life, some happy, some sad, and some intolerably painful. This was one such moment. My cry of joy could be heard in the hallway. Four months of effort, all distilled into one moment of pure joy, into a rubber stamp being pressed onto a medical form, into the long-expected "I have the doctor's approval."

I remember walking out into the sunny street and feeling the whole world smiling at me. I couldn't stop smiling back at it. I just walked down the street to my car and felt incredibly fortunate and blessed. I immediately called and set up an appointment with my family doctor. After all, for me the journey could not end until I saw him erase the permanent diagnosis from my medical record. The journey could not end until I received a printout from which that diagnosis was absent.

My family doctor, in contrast to the pulmonologist, was extremely reserved. Something prevented him from being joyful with me. I can't pretend I wasn't disappointed with his response. I had built up this moment in my imagination and now felt put down. I had entered his room waving the pulmonologist's form like a little girl might, almost chanting at him, "Told you so, told you so. I did succeed, and you were wrong!"

But what did this wet blanket do? Took the form, reviewed it briefly, muttered, "Okay," and then asked, "So what do you want to do?"

What do I want to do? What do I want to DO? I wanted to beat some sense into him, that's what I wanted to do. Instead, I just answered, "I want you to erase my diagnosis of asthma so it will no longer appear in any medical form with my name on it."

While he was fiddling with the computer and trying to identify what he needed to press in order to erase a "permanent diagnosis," I dared to ask him, "Doctor, aren't you happy for me?" I was not prepared to have anything or anyone overshadow my joy or the significance of that moment for me. As far as I was concerned, at that moment I was the cancer patient who had beaten cancer.

The doctor's stiff and detached mien didn't change in the least when he answered my question. "Of course, I'm happy for you. I just want to see how you are doing in the upcoming months." What he meant was that he didn't really believe that my affair with asthma was over yet. He had to see it with his own eyes, and "seeing with his own eyes" meant not seeing me in his clinic with an asthmatic seizure for at least a year. Only then would he allow himself to be happy, and only then would he share my excitement. Maybe.

It really took him a year, more than a year, to accept that it was all over. I saw him throughout the year because the children, God bless them, were running a viral and bacterial importation business from kindergarten and elementary school during that year, so our paths had occasion to cross.

He refused to believe I had cured myself from asthma for a long, long time. He saw me during the spring and fall of that year, saw me healthy, but his mind simply refused to believe his eyes. Those same eyes had seen me wheezing over so many years; his ears had heard my clogged-up lungs over so many seizures that he could not accept it was all over. Each time we met, he would ask me, "Well, how are you? Still well?"

He went so far as to take the initiative and question my husband about me whenever he saw him. "Say, is your wife really healthy? Are you quite sure she is not suffering any further seizures?" I wasn't angry with him. He was so used to a certain state of affairs, and suddenly something had changed for him all at once.

Finally, he got used to the new situation and accepted that I only showed up in order to receive referrals for blood assays to follow up about my thyroid gland.

As for me, success in my struggle with asthma gave me the inspiration to set out on another journey of self-healing.

Summary

To summarize, what did asthma teach me about myself?

- My soul neither forgot nor forgave the emotional hell, the humiliation and confusion I had experienced for so many years as a child and a teenage girl.
- I had to let go of my suppressed guilt for praying for the death of my father.
- I had an incredible amount of pent-up rage trapped within me that was burdening me and had to be released.
- I had to forgive my father in order to let go of the past.

CHAPTER 3
CHRONIC PAINS: MIGRAINES AND DISC HERNIATION

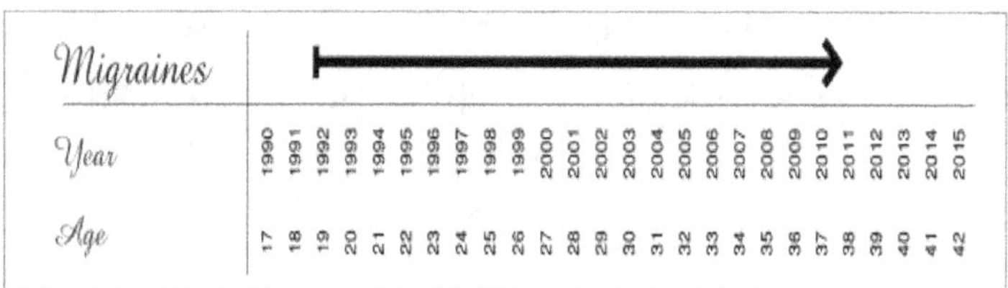

When I was eighteen, like a lightning bolt out of clear skies, my head was pierced by thundering pain. That was my first migraine, but it would prove to be only the first of hundreds of migraines that would arrive like unwanted guests in the chamber of my skull over the next two decades. In order to chase them out, I would swallow vast amounts of painkillers because the pain, that horrible pain, was so terrible, so indescribable.

For some reason, it took me several years to understand when exactly the pills should be taken to prevent this terrible pain, to preempt the migraine a second before it erupted, a second before the hammers began pounding my temples. Why? Because aside from the migraines, I also had "regular" headaches, and ibuprofen was good enough for them. I didn't want to consume the stronger pills if they weren't necessary.

Anyone who suffers from migraines knows that they usually don't show up at once, but that they evolve over several stages, gradually increasing in severity. Sometimes this can last several hours or sometimes only thirty minutes.

I didn't always know how long or how bad the pain would be, or why it occurred, so I often missed the window of opportunity to take the pill, and I wept when the wave of intense pain hit. There were many tears of pain and despair during this period of my life, and no, in case you were wondering, sitting in a dark, quiet room didn't help in the least. If anything, in my particular case, the silence and the dark just led me to focus even more on my pain and that focus intensified it.

To turn my mind away from the pain, I would often find myself staring at the flickering screen of the television, eyes half shut because it hurt to open them fully in the middle of a migraine episode. I stared absentmindedly at this or that stupid show, hoping that maybe, just maybe, the plot would be so fascinating I would be able to immerse myself in it until the pill kicked in and I would be back to my usual self.

Well, do you think that ever worked? Did I ever manage

to forget about the pain and dive into the imaginary world of the onscreen characters? Hell no. But I hurt more when I sat down in the dark and, every time the pain pounded at me again, I hoped that maybe this time it would help, maybe this time I would be able to fool the pain until the pills took effect.

Often, I ended up rushing to the hospital to receive medication that was stronger than the already powerful pills I was taking, after losing hope that the pain would pass away without medical intervention. Of course, I couldn't drive myself to the hospital when I was in the state that made a hospital visit necessary, so I found myself dependent on my husband and friends to get me there.

Usually the hospital would give me an injection in my behind, and my latest bout of migraines would be over after a merciful fifteen to thirty minutes. I would be back to myself and smiling again, and I would go on with my life as if nothing had happened. Until the next time. On rare occasions, I would get an intravenous injection of valium, and that was the best. Two minutes into the intravenous injection and my eyes would drift closed and serenity would replace the pounding pain. Hours of pain and suffering, all gone in a few seconds.

I always assumed that was what the heroin junkies you see in movies feel like—a needle in the vein and then fading away to a seemingly perfect bliss. That, at least, was how I felt when the valium blissed me out. I would go back home after the pain went away and then repeat the ritual a few days or weeks or months later, over a decade.

And then one day, the migraines just went away, never to return. More on that later.

THE SPINAL FRONT

When I was thirty, I suffered from disc herniation between the L4 and the L5 spinal vertebrae. A real classic in the world of disc herniation. What does this mean in simple terms? That the gel-like fluid inside the disc between these vertebrae had popped out of its casing. The results, for me, were insanely powerful back pains as well as pain projection to my outer thigh and calves and limitations to mobility occasionally accompanied by loss of sensation (paresthesia) in the feet. Oh, and also feeling utterly pathetic and handicapped.

How was that expressed in my particular case? Well, for two weeks, I was bedbound. Every expedition to the toilet required logistical planning that would put the D-day battle plans to shame, and their execution was literal Hell on Earth. So obviously, I sharply reduced my water intake in order to minimize these expeditions, and retained urine for hours and hours.

Still, wasn't lying in bed a chance to take a break from my hectic life and relax a bit? Not when I couldn't move, turn, or even cough or sneeze without collapsing in pain and frustration. I couldn't even help raise my children or comfort and be comforted by sharing a hug with them because it was all just too painful.

After two weeks, there was an improvement of sorts.

What does an improvement mean in the case of a slipped disc? It means you can leave the bed, walk around, move your body, even return to work at some point, but you learn to accept that the term "handicapped" now applies to you. You can't perform many movements, because it is too painful or because of the fear of pain (which is even more paralyzing than the pain itself). You can't pick up any heavy objects, not even little children who don't understand why Mommy won't pick them up and hug them anymore.

And while that pain might pierce the heart and not the nerve endings, it is just as fierce. You swallow a lot of pills that dim the pain for a short time, and your conversations become characterized by "Ouch!" spiced with "Watch out! My back!"

After long months of pain and visits to orthopedic specialists, who made clear that as far as they were concerned there was nothing to be done short of surgery, I eventually gave up and underwent a spinal surgery. By that point, I was in such a sorry and exhausted state that my fears of never waking up from general anesthesia, of waking up paralyzed, and all the other risks I had waived when I signed the consent form for the surgery couldn't hold me back from going through with it. I just wanted to get back to my life before the disc slippage, no matter what the price.

When the anesthesia started kicking in, I just kept on praying that the surgery would be successful with no complications. And then when I woke up, it seemed my prayers had been answered. I could feel, or more accurately not feel, relief from the ever-present pain in my back. A careful, probing movement to the right elicited no pain. The same with a movement to the left. A huge smile spread across my lips—the operation had succeeded! I could return to my normal life, I could smile again after so long.

And indeed, for a bit more than a year, I returned to my previous routine. All I had to deal with was steroids and inhalers for my asthma, painkillers for my migraines and, of course, the small matter of my bulimia, which I kept on concealing from the world. Inconsequential stuff like that. The smile came back to my face, my children were happy that their mommy was holding them in her arms again, and I returned to the gym, aerobics, and body-sculpting classes with a vengeance. I felt on the top of the world.

HERE WE GO AGAIN

And then, at the age of thirty-two, my disc slipped again, in the exact same spot where I had undergone the operation a year before. How did that happen? I fell out of an elevator. Well, to be more exact, I stumbled out of a malfunctioning elevator that opened its doors some fifteen centimeters below the building floor. I didn't fall badly or suffer any kind of open injury. I stopped my fall with my outstretched hands, but at that moment I knew something had happened because I could hear a gentle snap in my back.

My shame and embarrassment from the fall itself were greater than my concern at that gentle snap. "Why didn't you look where you were going, you foolish girl?" were the words that went through my mind as I looked left and right, making sure that no one had seen my embarrassing stumble. Then I picked up my scattered papers and ran off to the conference room for a meeting for which I was already running late. And yes, of course I used "I fell out of the elevator" as an excuse for my tardiness, even though I would have been late regardless. Wouldn't you do the same?

The meeting lasted more than two hours, and as it progressed I could feel my pain slowly increase, and I began to realize that something terrible was happening, something I had already thought I had put behind me, something that I had never dreamed, not even in my worst nightmares, would ever return. But return it did—my disc herniated. Again.

Do you know the saying "The surgery was successful, but the patient is dead"? In my case, it was "The surgery was successful, but the disc herniation is back." Immediately after the meeting, I told my colleagues that my back hurt from the fall, and I returned home. I knew deep inside that soon I would be unable to drive, and indeed that night I was in bed again in a state where every movement, right or left, was accompanied by hellish pains. The fact that my children had grown and no longer wanted me to pick them up was scant comfort. I had returned to feeling like the most miserable and pathetic woman in the whole wide universe.

This time I did not wait for months to submit to the surgeon's scalpel. On the other hand, nor was I really interested in undergoing another surgery with an unknown expiration date. Accordingly, while I was put under general anesthesia again, this time it wasn't for surgery. Oh no, this was just a minor surgical procedure. No forced entry, slicing and dicing, just some internal rearrangement of my willful vertebrae. And no new scars either, because the surgeon (in the "non-surgery") would use the old one as his entrance into my much-abused spine. I really hit the jackpot, in other words. Or at least that's how I reassured myself when the anesthesia kicked in.

Shall I tell you how wonderful I felt when I woke up? Well, actually things weren't that great this time around. Will I tell you that the pain had passed? Nope, not this time. Still, I was at least able to return to life as usual, right? Well, not exactly. What I returned to was to the life of a mild invalid, which was a bit like being "a little bit pregnant." What it meant was that the pain was bearable rather than unbearable, and I just had to learn how to live with it, because the alternative was to curl up in some dark corner and die.

I returned to mild exercise and general physical activity, constantly under the shadow of the fear that the wrong movement might result in another snap and then a rerun of two weeks of paralysis in bed, followed by months of horrible physical disability, pains, and helplessness. Just consider how many times a day you seat yourself, be it at a chair or a toilet, and understand how much space can be filled by fear of movement, which becomes your constant companion. That is how I, the terror of the pain, and the pain itself cohabited as bosom buddies for over four years.

And then one day, it stopped. One day, the pain just disappeared. I just didn't hurt anymore.

SO WHAT'S GOING ON?

As I said, the migraines also started one day and just disappeared. They were deleted from my operating system and were never reinstalled. In both cases, it took me several months to realize that my physiological-biological reality had shifted.

When did this change occur? Just a few months after I cured myself from asthma. But I can't put my finger on a date in my calendar and say, "Here, this is the day my back stopped aching. This is the day I stopped fearing migraines drilling new holes into my brain."

Why the difficulty? Because I was so busy with so many other things at the time. There were the various concealed disorders—the depressions and the hypermania attacks and the pills to balance them out. And, of course, my binge-eating and vomiting episodes, or the fact that I had started smoking weed in the early morning hours. Keeping all this concealed, my friends, takes up quite a bit of energy, and I will expand on that in the upcoming chapters.

The fact that I simply didn't notice that my back pains and migraines had ended is a deadly combination of a lack of basic self-awareness as a result of my euphoria from my "great triumph over asthma." This euphoria led me to plot out my next steps for the next campaign—getting my hypoactive thyroid gland back in order.

Yes, at that time Athena, the Greek goddess of war, and I were still best friends, and I defined everything in military-tactical-operational terms. I hadn't yet learned the importance of allowing space to learn of the journeys we undergo in this life, their twisted nonlinear courses, and the eternal truth they contain.

When did I remember to stop and realize what was happening? "Hey, I haven't been in physical pain for a long time. It must have been weeks since my back has ached and my head has pounded. What's going on here?" That founding moment came, as aforementioned, a few months after being cured from asthma.

So what happened? How did two different types of chronic pains that had been my constant companions over so many years suddenly disappear without me taking any active or deliberate steps to end them? Many years later, I found a detailed answer to that question that resonated with me in two fascinating books dealing with the curing of chronic pains: *They Can't Find Anything Wrong!* by Dr. David Clarke and Dr. John E. Sarno's *The Mindbody prescription: Healing the Body, Healing the Pain.* Each of them treated thousands of people who suffered from chronic pain, whose medical assays all showed no problems and for whom no pathological findings were found capable of pinpointing the sources or causes of the pains.

Dr. Clark speaks in his book about how mental stress creates those physical problems and even calls this stress the "invisible disease." He defines five categories of experiences that can result in illness: stress carried over from childhood, stress in the present, stress from trauma, stress from depression, and stress from anxiety. Each of these types of stress results in diseases or pains that cannot be explained in any other way.

Dr. Sarno (specializing in muscle-pain symptoms deriving from stress) explains in his book that rage in the subconscious portion of our soul leads to physical symptoms, with the rage itself deriving from three sources: rage from infancy or childhood that has never faded away, rage from stress we apply to ourselves (as in the case of people with a tendency for perfectionism or a desire to please others), and rage in response to real stress in everyday life.

These physical symptoms, he says, have a purpose, which is to prevent repressed emotions from emerging into consciousness by distracting us from the emotional world to the physical world. That is an avoidance strategy. The subconscious portion of our soul decides these deep memories are so dangerous or threatening to us that it represses them. The physical symptoms are actually part of a repression mechanism. In simple terms, you are better off dealing with the pain than with its source right now.

To summarize, both Dr. Sarno and Dr. Clark single out our souls and emotions as the sources of these chronic pains. Behind every pain they met as doctors, there was a hidden, underlying story, and as soon as the source of the mental tension or negative emotions was identified, the pains just passed, either immediately or after some time. But it was the awareness of the connection between body and soul that played a role in the process of healing the thousands of patients who reached their doorsteps.

So what happened in my case? Both my migraines and my back pains disappeared after I confessed, faced up to, and psychologically and spiritually treated my past as a battered child who experienced over many years stress and fear, as well as a conflict over my very identity. Was I a good person or a bad girl who deserved to be punished and beaten by her father?

During my therapy sessions and in the guided imagery session where I beat up my father, I vented out the repressed anger, the pent-up rage, the humiliation, shame, and helplessness that had become permanent parts of my emotional makeup. The transfer of the focus of consciousness from the physical to the psychological and dealing with the emotional-spiritual source of my pain meant that the physical symptoms of the pain became unnecessary, and therefore disappeared.

Unlike the migraines, which had shown up as soon as I'd left my childhood home, the disc herniation appeared later and demonstrated, on the physiological level, the terrible stress I labored under in the framework of the demanding advertising field I worked in for many years. For years, I felt that I didn't really have emotional support from my superiors. The daily stress was sometimes truly insufferable, and I frequently experienced situations in which I felt I was being backstabbed by colleagues and superiors.

I couldn't break away from this field for many different reasons, primarily but not exclusively financial, and I couldn't listen to myself and hear how I really deserved to be treated, so my body did it for me. It put me out of commission for weeks, and organized a time-out for me to recalibrate my systems and consider my place in life anew.

In retrospect, I can only say that I did not listen to

it or make proper use of the time it had provided for me. So my body repeated its message a year later and in a far harsher way—a disc herniation that was accompanied with a nervous breakdown (more on that later).

And what did I do when I recovered? I returned to the exact same field, because it was the path of least resistance, and my back pains returned to let me know that something in my life was wrong. Only when I finally treated myself properly (on my journey to heal my asthma) and when I finally looked inside myself, acknowledged what was, purified myself, forgave and accepted myself did something within me feel that the message was transmitted and internalized. Only then did the pains recede, disappearing without warning, just as they had appeared.

SUMMARY

To summarize, what did my chronic pains teach me about myself?

- The emotional-mental stress that I lived through in my childhood marked me on the physical level.
- For many years, I had repressed not only pent-up rage from my childhood but also stress that I had placed upon myself in the present by my high-demand occupation.
- I wasn't listening to myself. I was not recognizing my own needs.
- I must never allow people to treat me in a way that is not respectful or fair.

CHAPTER 4

HYPOTHYROIDISM: ROUND 1

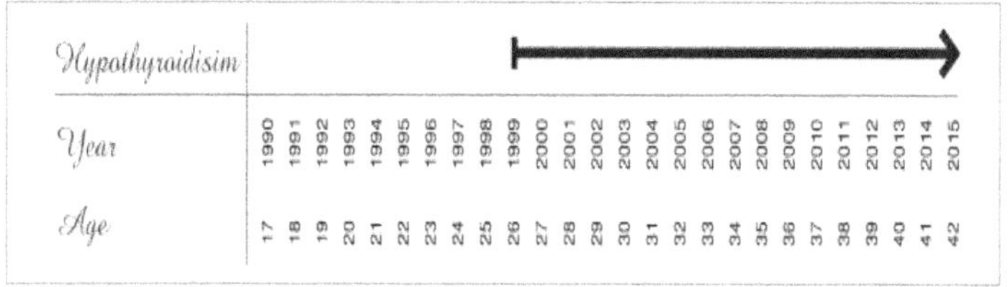

Why did I select my thyroid gland as my next objective following my victory over asthma? Mostly due to one simple reason: it was, at the time, the only disease I was not concealing from the world. It was a physical disease for which I was not, according to conventional medicine, responsible, and on whose account I needed not be ashamed any more than I would be ashamed of diabetes or rheumatism. Besides, I was not yet ready, not even close to ready, to give up smoking joints.

This was the second front of the seven campaigns I waged to be healthy again, and remained the most stubborn and hardest to resolve. It was the crème de la crème, the pinnacle of my journey, and the Holy Grail at the end of the road. This part of my journey had many interruptions and pauses along the way, but the way it first started is as follows.

The year was 2007, I was thirty-three years old, and I was in the endocrinologist's clinic, the one with the doctor specializing in the body's hormonal node (endocrine) system. I was also suffering from my first major depression and was already consuming copious amounts of steroids, psychiatric pills, and painkillers.

I arrived at the doctor because my blood tests had shown that my thyroid gland was not functioning properly. This was expressed in the kilograms I had gained, my afternoon exhaustion, and my irregular bowel movements. The thyroid gland regulates metabolism by producing a hormone called thyroxine. Low activity by the gland (for which the medical definition is hypothyroidism), is a situation in which the gland does not produce sufficient thyroxine so there is a considerable slowdown in the metabolic rate throughout the various systems of the body.

This is what leads to weight gain and obesity, chronic fatigue, irregular bowel movements, hair loss, disruption of menstruation, and even damage to female fertility. A whole whooping party of disruptions, and all of them can be traced to a single gland in the neck. This is often caused by an autoimmune disease called Hashimoto's disease in which the body's own immune system attacks the gland and destroys it.

"What happened to you in 1999?" the endocrinologist asked me in that first meeting, and I innocently answered that nothing special had happened to me in that year that I could recall. "Are you aware that your gland was hypoactive even then?" he asked me while going over data on the screen.

"What do you mean?" I snapped back without thinking. How could I have known this? Nobody told me or even hinted anything remotely like what he was telling me. "This can't be," I continued, aggressively deflecting his assertion.

"Are you arguing with the data on the screen?" he asked me in a reprimanding tone.

I answered at once that I was not arguing with him, but I could not understand how this data had showed up in my blood tests over so many years without any physician noticing or referring this anomaly to me.

"How can I know why no one else noticed this?" he shot back. "I am not responsible for what happened in the past. I know what I see in the system, and I see that in 1999, the measurements were already irregular. I can't tell what year this all started, because there is no earlier record of blood tests."

I was shocked. I literally found myself unable to respond, not something with which I was familiar. This is the place to explain that the primary parameter measured in regard to the thyroid gland activity is the TSH measurement. This stands for thyroid-stimulating hormone, whose role is to stimulate the thyroid gland to produce and secrete hormones. Its sound values range between 0.35 and 5.5 u/ml. A deviation upward indicates that the gland is not functioning properly, and therefore not producing the hormones that negatively regulate TSH production in the hypothalamus, leading to over-production of TSH.

Guess what my parameters were? 20.22 u/ml. Indisputably,

a very respectable deviation. I wasn't shocked by the deviant TSH levels; I was shocked that no one in the medical system had ever noticed it over so many years, even though I had undergone regular medical follow-up during both my pregnancies.

"Did you have any difficulties getting pregnant?" he asked.

"Not at all" I answered immediately.

"You had no problem getting pregnant for the second time?" he asked, surprised.

"No, no problems," I answered and tried my luck again. "Doesn't it seem odd that I went through two pregnancies but no one noticed that my TSH was so deviant?"

No luck. He grew irritated and grumbled, "I already told you that I don't know what happened."

"Why is this even happening?" I asked him toward the end of the first meeting, and he told me that there was no way to know, but that I was very lucky because the treatment was very simple and far more harmless than the steroids I was taking to treat my asthma.

"Just take one pill a day to get an artificial replacement for the hormone the gland is not producing enough of, and your body's balance will be restored," he said, trying to cheer me up.

"But until when will I have to take this pill? How long will it take my gland to work things out and return to proper functioning without external boosts?" I shot back, not really comforted by his words.

"Well, given the condition of your thyroid gland and the

fact that it has been malfunctioning for years, I do not see how you can stop taking the pill right now. But let's start and see how it goes and then move on from there," he answered with well-calculated caution and sent me on my way with a prescription.

I remember being very confused. On the one hand—joy! I'll take some pills and I will finally be able to shed the extra weight that had suddenly appeared, which I was simply unable to get rid of. On the other hand—what a bummer! More pills to add to the daily collection? Where had this all come from all of a sudden? And what about the next day and those that would follow? Would I be diagnosed with something else which would require even more medication?

But I had no choice, so I compartmentalized my confusion and began taking the pill. For the next three years, I played around with the dosages of Eltroxin under the supervision of the endocrinologist and bi- or tri-monthly blood tests. At first, I increased the dosage in order to see if that would help me lose weight, and then I experimented with the amounts and dosages because it gave me a type of control over my body and my health that I felt I had lost, and also because I really was curious to see what it did and find out how the change in dosage would be expressed. My endocrinologist was not pleased with my experimentation, to say the least, but I really didn't care.

SETTING FORTH WITHOUT SUPPORT OR ENCOURAGEMENT

Let's fast-forward a bit. The year is 2010, I am thirty-six and on my first steps on the journey of self-healing, right after my triumph over asthma and I am, once again, seated before my endocrinologist. But this time I am not bewildered. I am excited as I share with him my triumph over asthma and my grand plans to vanquish hypothyroidism and restore my thyroid gland to a full and sound function.

"Asthma is psychological, that is well known," he blurted out immediately, his face sealed as if to prevent even a fragment of my joy from penetrating. He added, "Hypothyroidism is different—you won't succeed."

For the second time in his clinic, I was shocked. At the speed in which he determined I wouldn't succeed, at his apathy when he said it, and the contempt he casually expressed toward my efforts over the past four months with his "Asthma is psychological, that is well known." If it was so well known that it is psychological, then why hadn't he told me so before?

"Why are you so sure I won't succeed?" I asked, trying hard to conceal my hurt feelings. Although I had always been taught that the way to avoid being disappointed was to not develop expectations, something within me still expected to receive a modicum of support and encouragement before embarking on my new path.

"It is true that asthma is psychological, as is proven by the fact that I eliminated it by treating its source, but why does this mean I cannot aspire to, and succeed in, repairing my thyroid gland?" I asked him.

I really didn't understand how he, who already understood that the source of one disease was emotional and that illness could be cured by treating the psychological origin of the disease, could say in the same breath that the thyroid gland simply could not be cured.

"I've heard about many cases of recovery from asthma, nothing special about it. But this is a much more complex case. The thyroid gland is responsible for so many functions and so many systems, you have no idea how complex it is. And in your case, it hasn't been working properly for many, many years, and you have been taking the pills for a few years already. Does it make sense to you that the thyroid gland would suddenly be restored to proper function?" he concluded his speech, looked at me and asked, "Do you understand me?"

I nodded but couldn't answer him verbally. He must have interpreted my silence as despair and therefore said more softly, "Look, it isn't that I don't want you to be healthy. What you did is really wonderful, but you need to understand that there is no recorded case in medical history of a thyroid gland under your conditions restoring itself to full self-functionality. There is no precedent for such a thing."

"So maybe I will be the first person in the world to make it work?" I asked in a whisper, making one last attempt to squeeze out something that might help me along the way.

"Sorry, you won't make it. Your effort is simply wasted," he answered and turned to his computer, a hint that our appointment was over.

"What if I get off the pills?" I asked while preparing to leave.

"Then you will be solely responsible for the outcome, and I strongly recommend against it," he answered in irritation. It was clear that I had used up what little patience he had to begin with for me.

FIRST CAMPAIGN

That day, I did not take my Eltroxin pill. I began to imagine how I would return to his room and wave my completely sound blood test form in front of his face, just like I had waved the Pulmonary Institute form. I spent two minutes every day imagining this scene, which might not arrive for many years to come, to the point of near despair.

A month after I got off the Eltroxin, I did a blood assay and panicked. My TSH was at 39.95. Almost double my level during all the years in which I was unaware of the disease and at the initial diagnosis. My measurements had leapt at once to nearly ten times their Eltroxin-medicated levels. My endocrinologist was also panicked at the result and called me in to read me the riot act.

"Do you see what comes of fooling around? You need to internalize that this is no game. You are inflicting harm on yourself." The meeting ended with strict orders to return to the medication at once. Reprimanded and with my tail between my legs, I went back on the Eltroxin, but I decided that I would no longer see this particular endocrinologist.

Although he was considered an expert in his field, he never really made me feel at ease and simply didn't create a pleasant atmosphere. He was apathetic and unpleasant, and I had had enough of that. I had lost my first battle big-time and internalized, in spite of my irritation at the endocrinologist being proved right, that this really wasn't as simple as the asthma.

Still, I refused to give up. I knew I had to find a source of positive energy to keep me charged up on the long road to the self-healing of my thyroid gland, even if I didn't even know where the road was or where it led. This doctor, I knew, could never provide me with that kind of energy.

Second Campaign: A Juice Fast

My second campaign against hypothyroidism started six months later, when I, then a journalist, was sent to cover a spiritual juice fast workshop lasting eight whole days. For those eight days, only organic vegetable juices were consumed, leaving the stomach in a state of total rest because there were no fibers in the juices. This gave the body time to cleanse itself from any toxins accumulated over the years.

In addition, energy that would usually be directed to digesting food would instead be channeled to sitting silently, meditating, and connecting to yourself and your higher being. I did not yet understand at this point what this meant exactly, but I felt that this was the positive experience I had been waiting for, especially since the supervisor of this workshop was an overseas doctor who was both a psychiatrist and international expert on nutrition and fasting and who had cured people all over the world from diabetes. He was also a very spiritual man and had written eight books on these topics. This man knew what he was talking about.

I let him in on my scheme to restore my thyroid gland, and to my very pleasant surprise he was not incredulous and did not rule out the possibility of success. He explained that success was possible but that, nonetheless, it would be a long path to walk and must be taken gradually, one step at a time. I couldn't wean myself completely off the pills, not all at once, and had to add to my diet additives for my gland and additional systems in the body, which were not found to be in an ideal state based on my blood tests.

I was encouraged by the experience, primarily because I finally felt that there was a professional who was listening to me and not treating my desire to cure myself as a silly, childish whim that would soon pass.

When the fast was over, I asked the doctor to examine me physically and to adapt the proper additives (vitamins, minerals) for my thyroid gland's recovery. It was the first time I had run into the use of kinesiology. In simple terms, this is a technique where the body is asked questions by stimulating a muscle and watching its responses. If we liken the mind to a computer with a massive databank, kinesiology enables access to the computer by using the muscle to provide us with the information we desire. The entire process is based on the assumption that the body does not deceive you like the conscious mind does, and that the body provides answers to issues that lie under the surface without being affected by conscious desires and/or manipulations.

Over the next few months, I was charged up with excitement again. I took all of the additives my body asked for in that examination, gradually reduced my Eltroxin dosages, and went back to imagining my triumphant return to the endocrinologist, waving the form with the sound blood tests under his nose. I even thanked myself daily for the courage to cure my thyroid gland each day.

But a few months later, I ran out of additives. I should, perhaps, mention that the additives this doctor recommended were extremely high-quality, and were therefore very expensive. The blood tests so far had not shown any significant change, and I had no funds available for another big purchase. My initial enthusiasm at resuming the campaign had waned and, following another disappointing blood test, the second campaign faded away, not with a bang but with a whimper.

"It's all right," I convinced myself. "So you are on a hypothyroid treatment pill. That isn't really all that bad; there are problems in the world that are far worse." Deep inside, I knew that my concealed eating disorder and manic-depressive disorder were far more serious problems.

THIRD CAMPAIGN: I ALSO WANT A MIRACLE

This campaign was initiated on a pleasant evening in October 2012, with a story that a friend who stopped by with her kid told me. That friend had been diagnosed with hyperthyroidism when she was young, and for years she was dependent, just like me, on Eltroxin to balance her metabolism.

The year before, a faulty Eltroxin batch scandal had broken out (see expansion box) and she was among those who had suffered from the side effects of the new pill. When the story broke in the media, she decided that this was a great opportunity to get off the pills.

Guess what? Nothing happened, no side effects whatsoever, and her TSH measurements stayed exactly the same without the pill.

"How can that be?" I asked, infected with maddened enthusiasm.

"I can't explain it," she answered. "I just kept feeling okay, as if nothing had changed. My first blood test, one month after I stopped taking the pill, showed the exact same TSH measurements as the previous one, and my second blood test two months later also showed TSH well within the norms, so I felt safe enough to return to my endocrinologist."

Yes. She, just like me, had experienced trepidation at the thought of what her endocrinologist would say.

"Well, what did he say? How did he respond?" I asked. My curiosity was killing me.

"He told me that if I had asked for his opinion before I had stopped taking the pill, he obviously would have advised against this course of action, but now that it was done, he was happy for me and just said I should continue tracking my TSH levels."

"That's it? You didn't ask him how this outcome was possible? How your thyroid gland could return to being functional after so many years?"

"He couldn't offer an explanation," she replied. And somehow, I was not surprised at her response. "He just said that sometimes things happened that medical science could not really explain, and the important thing was that I was well."

In October 2011, Israeli media exposed one of the greatest pharmaceutical scandals ever. This scandal centered on the pill given to treat hypothyroidism—Eltroxin. It seemed that the massive pharmaceutical company that had manufactured this pill over dozens of years had decided for reasons known only to it to change the formula of the pill. Not only had it done so without updating those concerned in an orderly and proper fashion, it continued marketing its product as usual, only in a new package.

When thousands of reports of severe side effects began coming in from patients in countries all over the world who had received the new formula, the company silenced them. Accordingly, when the new formula reached Israel in 2011, it was authorized for distribution on the fast track without any of the questions that were supposed to protect the patients receiving Eltroxin being asked. Israelis were not, of course, immune to the side effects. (It is estimated that two hundred and fifty thousand people in Israel received the medication.)

The media became aware of and exposed the problem when thousands of patients complained to their doctors that something was wrong and even set up forums to promote and increase awareness of the issue. This was a scandal on the scale of Remedia (a defective baby formula), but the fatalities in this case were mostly older people, whereas the young "only" suffered from severe side effects.

Even after the Eltroxin scandal was exposed in the media, the Israeli HMOs took months to provide their patients with pills from other manufacturers, and it was only in the beginning of 2012 that Eltroxin-dependent patients received relatively safe prescriptions. This was a blatant case of the patients' well-being not being the top priority of the medical system as a whole, let alone the pharmaceutical companies.

My friend's revelation was the opening shot of that campaign, and I went off the Eltroxin pill the very next day. That was on October 11, 2012. I remember telling myself that morning, all eager to go forth and do battle once again, "Remember this date." I remember saying to myself, "This is the last day of your life you will take Eltroxin."

I prayed for a miracle to come my way as well, for almost a month. "There is no reason to be ill and there is no reason to prevent myself from getting well," I encouraged myself twenty times a day. Then, at the end of that month, I took a blood test. My TSH level was 34.93. I gasped for breath in shock. What? How could this be? But I immediately restored my resolve and encouraged myself that while I had yet to get my miracle, this was only the beginning. I took a deep breath. I wouldn't let this disappointment steal my thunder. This was no more than the opening engagement of the campaign; there would be many more to come.

Congratulations, You're Pregnant!

As chance would have it (but nothing in life happens by chance, does it?), a few days after this setback I discovered, to my amazement, that I was pregnant. Again.

The bombshell dropped in my gynecologist's office. He looked at my blood test results and asked me, "What is this? Why are your TSH levels so high? This isn't normal."

"I stopped taking Eltroxin about a month ago, and that is why the levels jumped," I answered.

"Are you mad? You're pregnant!" he yelled. "Get right back on your pills. This is no time to be playing games. After you give birth, you can go back to this foolishness."

"But I made a decision to stop taking this pill, and I'm not going to take it anymore," I answered.

Utterly shocked at my answer, he fired back at me the most horrifying sentence I would hear in all of my campaigns. "If you don't intend to take the Eltroxin, you might as well have an abortion right now because your child will probably be born deformed."

In spite of all my preparations, I was unprepared for this answer. I felt like the campaign had been pulled out from under my feet and that I was falling. Deformities? What was he talking about?

He went on. "Do you understand what I am telling you?

There is another person you need to take responsibility for. This isn't just about you." And then he fired the final, fateful sentence. "I can't assume responsibility for the outcome of such an imbalanced pregnancy."

I will never know if he intended to say this sentence out loud or whether it was a thought that passed through his mind and was blurted out inadvertently. What I do know is that sentence immediately grounded me again, and as soon as I felt secure on my foundation, an inner voice told me, "He isn't the one taking responsibility. Only you can take responsibility."

And I just knew. I knew only I could take responsibility for my pregnancy and for my child, and that I couldn't expect anyone, certainly not an HMO doctor who must cover himself from future patient claims, to do it for me or instead of me. That is why I wasn't angry at him or the harsh things I heard from him.

But his anger had managed to shake me, which is when I remembered that my hypothyroidism had been present in my previous two pregnancies as well, but no one had shouted at me then, because no one had even noticed my condition, including this gynecologist. The fact was that I had already gotten pregnant twice, and easily, had sound pregnancies with no complications and gave birth twice, also with no complications. The children born had both been healthy, bouncing babies—not deformed in the least.

So why should the third time be any different? Why should I not have another standard pregnancy and give birth to a healthy child? Why should my current child be deformed? What has actually changed besides being informed? Nothing. On that day, I made the decision to stay off the pills and take full responsibility for my child.

EMPOWERMENT FROM OUTSIDE

I called a teratogenic consulting center to receive professional information. The center provided information and instruction for the general public and concentrated updated data from all over the world. Anyone could call and get free consultation from a doctor, because in this center the people answering the phones were all doctors. This was the best medical call center I was likely to find.

I spoke with a kind doctor for over forty-five minutes. She told me, in a calm and pleasant fashion, about the dangers unbalanced pregnancies like mine involve. I understood that the "deformities" my gynecologist was talking about, and which I understood to be physical deformities, were actually problems with cognitive development that arose in a later stage of the child's life, and that it was a risk, but not a certainty.

The defining moment for me was when the doctor explained that such risks also existed in perfectly standard pregnancies. In other words, there have been cases in the world where, even when the thyroid gland was balanced and in the normal range, similar cognitive problems developed among children. I needed no more than that. An inner voice cried out that some things were out of my hands and were written in Heaven, and this was the last nail driven into the coffin of doubts, misgivings, and fears.

Nonetheless, written in Heaven or not, the responsibility to do the maximum I could was in my hands, which is why I was assisted throughout the pregnancy by two additional medical professionals, who provided me with the support I needed during this period. The first was a chiropractor–kinesiologist and the second was a surgeon-homeopath. Each of them had recovered from a disease via unconventional methods, and each of them had assisted dozens of people in recovering from various diseases, including chronic ones.

The chiropractor played around with my vertebrae, as only chiropractors know how to do, and also queried my body about its needs in this pregnancy in terms of minerals and vitamins through kinesiology.

I came to him once a month, and each time he performed another kinesiological examination. I took all the additives the kinesiological examinations recommended, of which there were quite a few. They cost me thousands of dollars, as they could only be imported from overseas, but taking them resulted in positive effects on my blood tests. My TSH levels dropped from 34 to 20 during those months, which greatly encouraged and empowered me.

The kinesiologist also told me that he was able to help many women with hypothyroidism, but they mostly came to him after short periods of hypothyroidism, whereas in my case there was a long period of inactivity, which is why my recovery period would be longer.

The other doctor, my surgeon-homeopath, accompanied

me throughout the pregnancy, encouraged me, and reminded me that my infant and I were just fine. To his credit, he was the only one who dared (in his own way) to take responsibility. I emailed him the results of the blood tests and the specifications of the additives, and he reviewed them and occasionally provided advice and direction.

In the middle of June 2013, my fourth sweet child was born in a natural birth, bursting and squealing with health. Something inside me took a deep sigh of relief. I did it! I had given birth to a healthy child. I had managed to go through my entire pregnancy physically and mentally healthy with a hypo thyroid gland. I could cool down a little, rest, and unwind the stress that had hovered over me throughout the pregnancy in spite of the reinforcement and empowerment I received from the "other"and in spite of my own inner knowledge that everything was all right. At the end of the day, I was taking responsibility for the welfare of another human being, and this responsibility was with me 24/7. So I relaxed, took a deep breath, and gave myself in to raising my new and healthy baby.

THE FOURTH CAMPAIGN: NATUROPATHY

The fourth campaign was initiated in early November 2013, when I stood on my scale and had to admit that I had simply failed to return to my pre-pregnancy weight, as I had done in my three previous pregnancies.

In my yoga class, I met a naturopathy doctor, who told

me as we were getting dressed in the locker room that she specialized in hormonal problems and women. The belief at the base of naturopathy is that the human body is capable of healing itself, and so the naturopath aids the body in healing itself using various gentle methods such as improving nutrition and treatment with medicinal herbs, nutritional additives, and etheric oils.

She told me that the bottom line was that my thyroid gland could certainly be balanced with the special formulas she made, and my inner voice cried out to me from within, "Go to her! Go to her! This is no coincidence, she can help you." I needed no further encouragement to get my ass in gear and embark to the front of another campaign.

For almost six months, I learned from the naturopath about proper nutrition in general, and thyroid-gland supporting nutrition in particular. Farewell to the entire Brassicaceae family of vegetables (cabbage, cauliflower, broccoli, turnips), and hello (as well as a first introduction) to many different kinds of seaweed, shellfish, and saltwater fish that contain relatively high levels of iodine (an extremely important mineral for the proper function of the thyroid gland and the production of relevant hormones). I drank special syrups twice a day made from special medicinal herbs that were specifically brewed for me, and even took a few additives she recommended.

In parallel, in another apartment in the city, I slowly learned—together with my spiritual teacher—about the features of my spirit and how they had contributed to form a physiological reality of a malfunctioning thyroid gland over so many years.

Throat trouble, I learned, is always related to deprivation or to difficulties in self-expression. Things that should have been said but were left unsaid for various reasons. I would have to learn to merge the desires of my eternal spirit with those of my temporal human soul, and from that unity would come true recovery and health.

If you are confused by my definition of the soul as temporal, and the distinction between spirit and soul, allow me to use this chance to take a small detour and explain. Briefly, as human beings, we live eternally as a spirit—we have a soul, and we dwell in a body. When we try to envision who we are—who we really are—we think of our mind, our conscience, our emotions, and our will.

Everything we experience in this life shapes, and is shaped by, our soul. When we will something to happen, it is our soul that provides that will. The soul is the story of us—but it is not the whole story. When our life ends, and before it begins, there endures the truly eternal part of us— our spirit. It too has desires, which shape the life we live, what we encounter within it, and how we react to it. If those desires conflict with what our personality—our soul— wishes, then imbalance and illness follow. What my spiritual guide was telling me was that I had to go beyond listening to my soul. I also had to attune myself to the desires of my spirit and resolve the conflicts between its agenda and the desires of my soul.

But what the hell did that actually mean in terms of things to do? Many questions for which I did not yet have answers troubled my mind, and the unknown was greater than the known. On April 2014, after about six months, I had a blood test. All of my efforts yielded a reduction from 36 to 26 and no more. I was terribly disappointed with the result. All of my efforts—including abstinence from cabbage, cauliflower, and broccoli—and that was it? My disappointment led me to drop out of the race again. I had to give it a rest for a while.

A FIFTH AND FINAL CAMPAIGN

In December 2014, I recharged myself with the proper sources of energy, and the will to be healthy again reemerged from the dank dungeons where it had languished over the previous six months. The trigger this time was a multisensory meditation course by a spiritual teacher who taught us how to use meditation as a tool to connect to ourselves rather than to detach from this world and escape into others.

I began practicing meditation on a daily basis, and in its framework, I also imagined repairs to my thyroid gland and thanked it for the lesson it was forcing me to learn. In addition, I performed a wide variety of various energetic treatments on myself that I had learned about in additional courses that year.

On January 2015, I decided to check out how all of my energetic work had affected my chemistry and took another blood test. It showed that my TSH had descended from 36 to 24.91. I was disappointed again with the very limited improvement, and the wind began to leave my sails. I found myself unable to maintain the intensity or frequency of the energetic treatments and was left only with the daily meditation.

In February, I took more blood tests, and saw that my TSH had climbed back up to 30.09. I finally broke down for good and accepted the fact that being balanced for all practical purposes without the pill was good enough. I wasn't gaining weight, my bowel movements were regular, and most importantly, not only was I not tired, I was filled with good energy all day and was happy.

So I couldn't achieve the impossible with my thyroid gland. But hey, I comforted myself, I had done the impossible with my four other diseases: asthma, manic depression, bulimia, and drug addiction. I had also gotten over two different types of chronic pains that had been my companions for many years.

"Isn't that an achievement I can take pride in?" I asked. "Damn straight!" I reminded myself that I had achieved my overarching goal—a transition from a young girl collapsing under the weight of pills she was hooked on to a slightly more mature girl who was living a pill-free existence. Game over. I had won by points, six to one.

CHAPTER 5
BIPOLAR DISORDER

Bipolar Disorder																										
Year	1990	1991	1992	1993	1994	1995	1996	1997	1998	1999	2000	2001	2002	2003	2004	2005	2006	2007	2008	2009	2010	2011	2012	2013	2014	2015
Age	17	18	19	20	21	22	23	24	25	26	27	28	29	30	31	32	33	34	35	36	37	38	39	40	41	42

My bipolar disorder was not something I was born with. Like many of my other chronic diseases, it just broke out in my early thirties without any early warning. The psychiatrist who had treated me over the years hated the term manic depression, which was more common because, in his words, "The medical profession stopped using this term twenty-five years ago." But it doesn't really matter what you call it. The bottom line is that the disorder transformed me from a bubbly, smiling, optimistic, energy-filled, and zesty woman to a wreck marooned in deep depression.

And when I say deep, I mean very deep. Just to keep things interesting, the depressions were interspersed with hypomanic attacks (an uplifted mood and "high" type behavior but without loss of judgment). It was expressed in my case as nonstop chatter over several days until I was hoarse. I couldn't stop speaking nonsense, and I felt like James Bond, one second before conquering the world.

My first depression came at age thirty, when I decided to withdraw from the field of advertising where I had been employed for quite a few years in order to find myself. After spending two months at home, my mood began to sink and I found myself in a dark place. I didn't want to leave bed in the morning, I had no energy to spend time with my children, and I didn't feel like seeing people at all, not even good friends. No one.

At some point, a family decision was reached that it would be better for all concerned for me to go back to doing what I knew best, and I returned to advertising after six months at home. Very quickly, my depression declined and I was back to myself, back to the happy and smiling person I used to be.

Eighteen months later, in a new workplace, I had my stupid fall from the elevator (which I described in chapter 6 in the disc herniation section), which kept me bedbound for two weeks. I went back to work at once, but what I went back to was the chaos of a nonstop crisis mode. On top of all that, I was still suffering from terrible back pains.

At some point, anxieties came calling at my workplace and I began to be afraid of the most ridiculous things. Simple, routine tasks that I had performed for year with closed eyes suddenly seemed to me terribly frightening and impossible to perform. Even when I was told what to do, the anxiety drove my brain's neurons crazy, and I couldn't internalize what I was being told. Add to that the fact that I didn't fall sleep until 2:00 a.m. because I spent from midnight until that time clearing non-urgent mails that I couldn't get to during the workday. Then I would get up two hours later, at 4:00 a.m., terrified that I couldn't get to everything. You can guess what the pressure and lack of sleep led to.

The Breakdown

After two such inhumane months, the big day came. The day of the nervous breakdown, which led me to sink into such a deep depression that it made the one that preceded it look like no more than a small free sample of the shape of things to come. The day began as usual, with insane levels of stress and my heart beating like a drum before I even entered the office. Around ten o'clock, while I was trying to take control of a truly insane number of tasks, I received an email from an unsatisfied client.

I remember staring at the email, glancing at the endless list of tasks that lay before me, looking back at the email, and then back again at the list, unable to stop until my heart began beating loudly and painfully. That was the point where I felt I was losing it and that there was simply nothing I could do, not even breathe.

I went out for a smoke, but it didn't help as it usually did. I just couldn't breathe properly, and mostly I couldn't think a single coherent productive thought. I guess this was all apparent on my face, because the manager of one of the departments asked me if I was all right. I told him I wasn't feeling well and that something bad was happening to me. He walked me to my office while supporting me, helped me to my chair, and looked over my to-do list. Then he began talking to me trying to find out which fires to put out first.

At the moment he talked to me, an inner voice screamed in my head in an endless loop, "I can't, I can't, I just can't," for nearly two minutes. I simply couldn't take in any more external input. My receiver had burned out. No input and no broadcasting, either. At some point, my inner voice was externalized, and I began muttering, "I can't, I just can't, I just can't."

Only then did he realize that I wasn't with him, understand what was happening to me, and say, "Leave it, we'll manage. I'm taking you home."

Yes, it was an unbelievable faux pas for people to see me break down like this, but I was in such an unbelievably terrible condition that I no longer cared what people thought or said about me. All I wanted was to get the hell out and never come back. My nerves were so exposed and sensitive and pained that I had to minimize contact with the world.

My manager brought me home by cab because I wasn't in a condition fit to drive, called my husband to update him about what was going on and that I was home, told me several times that it would be okay and that I just had to get some rest, and returned to the office. He was my saving angel on that day and did what I was unable to do for months for a thousand different reasons. He got me out of the inhuman madhouse I was in and brought me back to the only place that I could exist or survive, my bed.

I didn't leave the bed for a week and didn't communicate with anyone. I simply couldn't. About a week later, a phone call came from a good friend. My sorry state had given her the courage to share with me that she had experienced something similar. She was being treated by a psychiatrist who was a great deal of help to her and she was taking pills that had helped her put a smile back on her face.

I was shocked. She had always seemed so happy and cool, so it was difficult to accept what she told me and match it with how I perceived her until this conversation. I found out that I wasn't the only one, that many people like me suffered from anxieties and depression. Not for nothing is depression known as the plague of the twenty-first century. Most people are simply too ashamed or scared to admit it or share it with others.

RECOVERY AT THE PSYCHIATRIST'S CLINIC

In March 2006, I arrived at my first meeting with the psychiatrist who would accompany me for many years to come. He put me on Seroxat, a drug from the SSRI family of antidepressant medications such as Prozac and Cipralex, which are better known to the public. These medications act on the neurotransmitter serotonin, one of three neurotransmitters found to be linked to mood disorders.

The psychiatrist explained that Seroxat has side effects such as headaches (no big deal, I was suffering from migraines anyway), insomnia (no big deal, it's not like I was sleeping well anyway), changes in appetite (never mind, I wasn't eating well anyway on account of my depression), feelings of fatigue (no big deal, I was spending all day in bed as it was), and a few other choice physical symptoms. The side effect that caught my attention the most and accompanied me for years to come was harm to sexual function. In other words, farewell to my libido—I look forward to meeting you again when I'm back to life off the antidepressants.

Well, all this was pretty darn bad, but being depressed was even worse. My psychiatrist also explained that he believed aside from treatment on the physiological-neurological level, I also required psychological therapy. So in addition to the medical treatment, I started therapy with a lovely psychologist. This lasted five months, until I decided I had gotten all the good that I could out of it.

In retrospect, it is clear that I wasn't really prepared to delve into the darker corners of my soul since I wasn't even able to reveal that my father had beaten me as a child (just a minor detail I neglected to share). Still, the combination of pills and therapy helped me return to my usual self—for a while, anyway.

So Let's Conceal It

A few days after that first meeting with the psychiatrist, I was back to work, with my mood showing some improvement. This was also when I first put on my "double concealment mask." I concealed my depression and nervous breakdown from everyone, and also the fact that I was on "mental patient" pills. I didn't want anyone to know that I was not well or think I was mentally unstable. This wasn't a comfortable situation, to say the least. I didn't know whether I was mad, mentally ill, or just out of balance. Whatever I was, there was no way that I could tell any of my family, friends, neighbors, or colleagues that I was on these pills. No way. Come to think of it, my concealment mask was a triple, not a double, since I was still concealing my bulimia as well.

And that was the start of a four-year period during which I experienced a roller coaster of highs and lows, mostly because every time I took the pill and stabilized, I immediately stopped taking it because I felt bad and didn't feel like I needed it or wanted to take it anymore. At some point, the psychiatrist switched me to Cipralex, which was not as strong as the Seroxat.

In those years, I grew and progressed in my second career as a journalist, a career I really loved and that felt more right. We also moved to a large house that we built from scratch. I had our third child, and life was seemingly perfect.

But it wasn't. Not really. Because this imbalance overshadowed all the good things that happened. This was made worse by the extreme transitions between depression and hypomania episodes due to the game I played nonstop with the pills: taking-improving-stopping-dropping, or rising-taking, and so forth.

My concealment of this imbalanced psychotic mess just

made things worse. Believe you me, concealment takes up a great deal of energy due to the steps required to maintain it and the simple fact that you are concealing secrets. Also, let us not forget that a concealment was occurring on both the bipolar and bulimia fronts. In short, it was fun, fun, fun. Still, I was optimistic and remained smiling and happy. Until one day I wasn't.

I WANT TO DIE

In the summer of 2010, I experienced what I would later call "my last great depression," which lasted four whole months. Like many of my depressions, it had nothing to do with anything occurring in external reality because my reality was, on paper, great in every respect—the personal, the professional, and the parental, as well as with my better half.

But still I sank into a depression that made all of my other depressions look like minor affairs. Why am I so decisive in my definition, do you ask? Because in this depression I really reached rock bottom—I wanted to die, to cease to exist. Yes, I literally wanted to die. Every morning when I woke up, I felt sorry that I had not passed away during the night, that God had not collected my soul back to his repository in the world to come. Because I was definitely sick of my time in this world.

I was done with it. Every breath I took was hard, and there was not a single minute in any day when I did not experience in my heart the depths of the abyss and the darkness that surrounded me. Whenever I drove somewhere, I would pray incessantly, "Please let a truck just run me over and end this terrible pain."

On less terrible and suicide-thought-prone days, I would offer a slightly more optimistic prayer along the lines of "May a truck run me over and injure me badly enough that I will have to be hospitalized in isolation for six months or so, during which I won't have to see anyone or talk to anyone or treat anyone." Something in my mind just changed and transformed the way I saw the world—and the concept of life in this world—to a nightmare.

This dark period brought me to a place where I first understood my brother-in-law, who had committed suicide a few years earlier at the age of thirty by jumping off the roof of a building. He too had suffered for many years from a severe bipolar disorder and then one day, when his suffering was just too terrible, he climbed up to the top of a building and leapt to his death in order to end it. I arrived at a place where I understood him and even envied him for no longer suffering.

All of a sudden, I developed an understanding of and sympathy for suicidal people in general. I understood their pain and the depth of their emotional-psychological anguish. Regardless of the specific circumstances that led them to make their decision, each of them had a personal story in which their choice to end their pain, and the reasons they simply could not go on, and escape to a place where they felt nothing ever again was understandable.

SUNRISE

My condition brought me back to the psychiatrist, who prescribed me a new pill named Effexor. My dosage started at 175 mg a day, but since I showed no improvement, it quickly rose to 250 mg a day. In spite of the high dosage, it took two months for the pill to start to work and affect my mood, even though it was supposed to kick in after one or two weeks. Something within me, deep within the depths of my subconscious, would not allow the pill to take effect and improve my condition.

Consciously, I may have been screaming for an alleviation of my condition, begging to feel better, crying out for the darkness to be banished from my life. However, as I later learned, our conscious is not really in the driver's seat; it is just the part of our mind that thinks it is. That is far from the truth.

Still, one day the pills did finally kick in and the sun shone in the sky once again. Life was back to being fun and thrilling and full of possibilities. I was smiling again, and I returned to being a functioning mother to my three children and a wife for my husband, who took a deep sigh of relief and was happy to tear off and incinerate the nurse's uniform that the situation had forced upon him.

That happiness lasted for no more than eight months, until May 2011. Those of you who have been taking notes may remember that this was when I had arrived at the juice fast workshop and decided I would stop taking my hypothyroid treatment Eltroxin pills. Again. Those eight months were, as of that period, the longest period in which I had taken antidepressants without on-again, off-again games. The trauma from that depression and the fear of returning to the dark places to which I had descended in its wake echoed for a good, long time and drove me to swallow my pill daily like a good little girl.

CHURCHILL WAS ALSO BIPOLAR

In the spring of 2012, I arrived at the psychiatrist because I wanted to get off the pills, only this time under his professional supervision, and he had a surprise waiting for me. He told me that I was suffering from a bipolar disorder. So where's the great surprise? Especially after years of therapy? Well, as fate would have it, the specific psychiatrist treating me was one of the rare professionals who was not fond of categorizing his patients by disease. Accordingly, he usually avoided giving a specific name to any disease or mental condition from which I suffered. A woman is defined by more than being bipolar; she is first of all a human being.

After having watched me for years in my waves of repeated mood swings, he had decided to share an orderly diagnosis with me in order to recommend a more fitting medical treatment for my condition. Over the years, we had spoken in terms of highs and lows, in terms of changes in my moods. He would tell me of an engine nozzle that would snap out of a balanced position, and this was enough for me. He also continuously repeated the mantra that the imbalanced chemical celebration in my brain was a hereditary, congenital condition, and that there was nothing to do about it besides provide a proper medical treatment.

Even when I had shared the successful psychological treatment that led to my recovery from asthma, he remained adamant. While sincerely happy for me, he explained in the same breath that my problem was not psychological but chemical, and that there was no non-chemical way to restore my balance. There was therefore no point in contemplating a balanced life without pills.

On that fateful day on which I received a title for the disease from which I suffered, he explained to me that the bipolar disorder had but one effective treatment, and that was the provisioning of a stabilizer. Just like antibiotics were the way to slay bacteria-causing infections of the lungs (pneumonia) and ibuprofen was how the side effects such as fever and pain could be relieved, the cure for bipolar disorder was a stabilizer such as lithium, while the ibuprofen-type relievers were Effexor or Cipralex.

My psychiatrist tried to comfort me by telling me that throughout history, many famous people had bipolar disorders, yet they nonetheless had left their marks upon the world. These individuals included Beethoven, Winston Churchill, Tolstoy, Van Gogh, and even Buzz Aldrin, who had traveled to the moon and back.

I left the meeting not knowing how to think or feel about the news. I had come to ask about getting off Effexor, but instead left with a recommendation to take lithium. What did the drug that Kurt Cobain, the Nirvana singer, had written his famous song about have to do with me? What did the medication that the movies showed as being given only to the most deranged individuals, turning them into apathetic and nearly robotic creatures have to do with me? This was the creativity killer of artists, wasn't it? That's what all the movies showed anyway.

My psychiatrist told me to think it over, that nothing was urgent, and that I should come back with an answer. Instead, I came back with a husband, who was rather more alarmed than I was with the doctor's prescription and wanted to hear what this was all about straight from the horse's mouth.

As for myself, my inner voice was screaming, "No way are you taking that drug! No way, absolutely none," and everything restated in this meeting did not stop me from reaching the conclusion, by myself, that whatever might happen, lithium was one line I was not prepared to cross.

When the Student Is Ready, the Teacher Reveals Herself

And so a number of months passed in which I stayed on the Effexor and gracefully ignored any recommendations that I move on to lithium, until November 2012, when I discovered (surprise!) that I was pregnant with my fourth child. The pregnancy gave me the courage I needed to get off the Effexor.

It completely nullified the fear that had prevented me from getting off the pills in the past, since I knew that as long as I was pregnant, I would not sink into depression. A pregnant body is a body that contains another life within it, and the presence of the additional life within me filled me with joy. What happened after the pregnancy was not important to me at that time. "I'll deal with the monster across the river after I cross the bridge," I told myself.

On May 2013, when I was eight months pregnant, the additional help I need appeared in the form of a spiritual teacher. This teacher was also a channeler, and for those of you who have no idea what that means, I'll say, in the simplest words I can think of, that someone who channels forms a bond with intelligent entities that do not reside in a human body, in order to receive and pass on information meant to help either a specific individual or humanity as a whole.

I summarized the eighteen months of weekly meetings with her as "psychological treatment for my spirit," which also helped light up, visualize, and clean out the shadowed portions of my soul, and eventually led to the unification of the desires of my temporal soul and the eternal spirit.

This, to make a long story short, is the advantage of the treatment I underwent in regard to a conventional psychological therapy that treats an individual as being composed of two parts, body and mind, that carry out a dialogue with each other and reciprocally affect each other, including through moods and diseases.

The trouble was that the psychological therapy lacked the third component of the human whole. That part is the eternal spirit. Wise people from different cultures and places on the planet understood, thousands of years ago, that man was composed of three parts: an eternal spirit, a temporary body, and the soul, which is also temporary, and bridges and mediates between them. If we ignore such an important component of the human equation, we can never solve it or understand it.

As soon as I began asking questions such as "Who am I? What am I? Why am I? What do I really want?" and understanding the contours of my spirit and its purpose in donning the temporary mask that is me, and all its complex, painful, and often ill biography, I discovered the reasons for the imbalance I experienced in my life throughout so many years, which was expressed on both the spiritual and physiological-chemical level in the brain. And as soon as I discovered those reasons, I seemingly magically found my balance again. I allowed my entire body to respond to the spiritual-mental processes that this investigation initiated and resonated with.

Gone With the Wind

So what did I get out of all this spiritual mumbo-jumbo? My greatest gain was the elimination of my greatest fear. As soon as my perception of death as the final end to all things lost its power, my fear from the great unknown disappeared along with it.

The second gain was ending my period of concealing my disorders from the environment. When we are ashamed of something we do or did, we conceal it, suppress it, and/or lie about it. But we cannot cure something we hide or fail to admit. When I began to understand and accept the fabric of my life and the reasons for everything that happened, shame began to fade away on its own.

This process enabled me to accept myself and all of my aspects, light and shadow. As soon as we accept who we are, shame disappears. When we stop feeling ashamed, concealment ceases. When concealment ceases, then it is possible to identify, talk about, and work on solving the problem.

The third thing I gained was the de facto end of my mood swings. Once I reached my spirit, recognized it, bonded to it, learned about it and its desires—and learned to integrate those desires with those of my temporal soul and all of its desires, flaws, and virtues—I returned the entire system to a state of permanent balance. As soon as my system was balanced, I suffered from no more extreme mood swings.

What about that supposed hereditary and congenital condition my psychiatrist had insisted upon for years? That same chemical problem in the brain that had led my neurotransmitters not to work properly? Well, that supposed congenital condition seemed to be simply "gone with the wind."

SUMMARY ON THE PSYCHIATRIST'S COUCH

In May 2015, I returned to my psychiatrist in order to fill in the blanks of my medical history, as sort of a background study before writing this book, but mostly for closure. I had not seen or spoken to him since November 2012, since I had gone off the pills.

"Doctor," I asked, "I want to know just how many bipolar individuals you have treated over the years who managed to get well and stabilize themselves without medication?"

"If you are referring to your own case," he answered, "you went through pregnancy and childbirth, which is a very positive event that involves hormonal changes. That's one factor. The other is getting off the steroids and other medications you were taking that were not related to your bipolar disorder, which are known to have a very bad effect on the neurotransmitters and the nervous system. The third factor is the psychological angle. In my opinion, spiritual or religious commitment can act as a substitute for cognitive psychological treatment."

His answer pissed me off. Why was this the first time he was telling me about the adverse effects of combining medication? I had been his patient for years and he knew about my other medical conditions, yet he had never raised the issue of cross-reactivity between the medications and their negative effects on my nervous system.

"Is that how you summarize my healing?" I asked, trying not to allow my irritation to take over our dialogue.

"I am afraid a bipolar disorder is primarily a chemical

problem with neurotransmitters and not greatly affected by psychological attitude or other factors. It's a hereditary, congenital condition," he said, again decisively and without any apparent doubt.

I repeated my question. "How many bipolar individuals have you treated over the years who managed to get well and stabilize themselves without medication?"

"My answer is that one of two possible things occurred." He answered, "Either I was wrong in my diagnosis or no one had ever done it before. That is my answer."

On the one hand, his answers did not satisfy me, but on the other hand, I was happy. I was the only one of hundreds of bipolar disorder patients the dignified doctor had seen over all the years of his career who had stabilized themselves without pills. I felt special, and I knew that he couldn't identify the factor that changed my condition from congenital-hereditary to nonexistent. I let go of him, together with my illness, with a rush of love.

SUMMARY

To summarize, what did my bipolar disorder teach me about myself?

- I hadn't listened to myself and I had allowed people and situations to divert me from what was right for me.
- Understanding the reasons and goals for which my spirit donned the temporal mask that was me, and the connection to both, restored my spiritual, mental, and physiological systems to a state of balance.
- Accepting myself and all of my aspects, both shadow and light, reduced my shame and eliminated my need to conceal my difficulties from others.
- Unifying the desires of my temporary soul with those of my eternal spirit led to serenity, acceptance, and relaxation, and eliminated the bipolar disorder from my life.

CHAPTER 6
BULIMIA

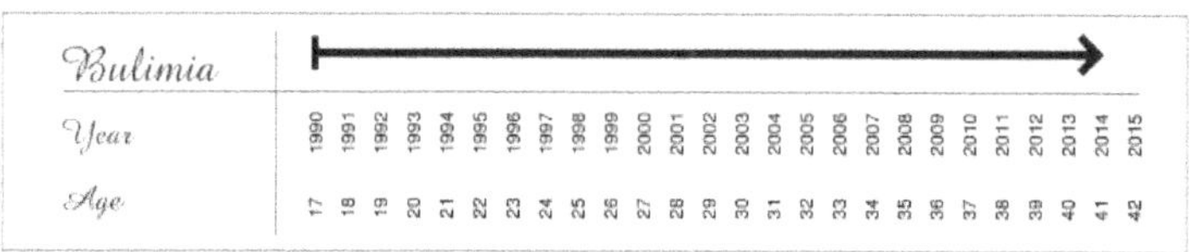

The first time I shoved a finger down my throat, I was seventeen and a half, which is about as cliché as you can get. I had read an article about a model who spilled the beans about how she had thrown up by pushing her fingers down her throat to keep her stomach flat before a fashion show. I read it and told myself, "Well, that's worth a try." It seemed like a simpler way to lose weight than a painstaking diet where I would have to consume massive amounts of lettuce.

Do you think it was easy? Hell no. It took me a few good tries to throw up properly. After all, it isn't like there is a manual for the novice vomiter—no precise instructions and no one to ask. It would be pretty embarrassing to approach someone for instructions on proper techniques for vomiting, don't you think?

The whole sorry business operated on experimentation,

mistakes, and wonderment. One, two, or three fingers? How deep? With or without drinking? How much can one eat before vomiting? Is it better to eat small helpings and vomit several times, or eat a great deal and vomit it all out at once? What is more practical? Does vomiting make noise or not? How much? Can they hear me from the other side of the door or not? How do I know that I vomited it all out?

In short, a great deal of questions that only extensive vomiting experience can answer and enable adaptation and calibration for the purposes of the user. I remember that I even went out once or twice in the evenings to throw up outside the house, in order to perform experiments in a safe, protected area "without any hostile forces" to deal with. We lived in a farm (at a *moshav*, a collective agricultural community), and each house had a plot of land an acre or more around it. There were plenty of places to throw up quietly without running into anyone or having anyone run over the contents of my stomach the next day.

Over the years I had become a true mistress of vomiting, and more importantly, in concealing the traces and covering my tracks. Do you think it is simple to vomit your guts out in residences shared with other people? Nothing could be further from the truth.

In public places, it is relatively simple. You don't know anyone and no one knows you. Nor is anyone keeping tracking you, and they don't really care about what you do behind the restroom doors. Go in, vomit, go out. Simple.

In private residences, on the other hand, it is much more complex to hide the vomiting, but those technical obstacles can be overcome with a little imagination, planning in advance, and particularly a fierce urge to vomit out your soul that takes over your entire essence and leaves you with no choice but to vomit.

I'll give you a few examples and principles to follow. Women, never vomit while wearing eyeliner or mascara; it smears and makes it very hard to conceal what you are doing. Lipstick is easy to fix. Eyeliner is more complicated, and I often found myself replying to the question "What happened to you?" with the answer "Smoke from my cigarette accidentally got into my eye and I rubbed it."

Always double-check at the entrance to a restroom whether it has an odor-prevention spray. There is a massive difference between a restroom with spray (yes, yes, yes) and one without (maybe, maybe, maybe). Often it is better to give up the vomiting itself because it's strong and the distinctive smell will be clearly apparent. Experienced vomiters should perform the spray check as soon as they arrive at the scene, even before the food itself, then match the amounts of food to the situation.

Another preliminary inspection, which is an absolute must, is to flush the water in the toilet *before* you do your business to get an idea of the flushing power. Strong or weak? Fast or slow? From personal experience, I strongly recommend against vomiting in a restroom where the flushing current is slow and weak. While this only happened to me once or twice—one time is enough to traumatize you. Either the vomit does not flush down (what does flush down is years of your life as you hysterically wonder how you found yourself trapped in a vomit-filled restroom), or the vomit floats on the surface of the toilet water, together with your anxieties and shame.

If possible, particularly in your own home rather than when you are guests in another home, it is recommended that you first vomit, then flush before voiding yourself. You are killing two birds with one stone that way. You gain enough time for the distinctive redness that vomiting induces in your eyes to pass (minimization of suspicious evidence), and leave the expected smell from a restroom visit behind you rather than that of vomit.

Let us also not forget the issue of timetables. Bulimia requires a complex multiparameter system of various timing calculations. When is the right time to vomit in terms of the location and number of people in it? How much time will pass before I am in a place where I can vomit? And subject to all of these calculations, the eating program itself is determined—what, how much, and when to eat—yes, it all revolves around the selected location and timing of your vomit's date with the toilet bowl.

CAUGHT IN THE ACT

Tired of all the vomiting stories? Well, just imagine how it is to live that way for years, what keeping all these dealings secret involves, how much energy is wasted on all this business and its mad concealment from the environment, and how many lies all this generates.

All means are fair to avoid getting caught, and what is surprising is that in all these years, I was only caught in the act once. It was in the army, in the clinic where I served as a medic, and the person who caught me in the act was one of the medics who served in my unit. He entered the lone toilet booth in the clinic after I had done my business and saw all the vomit there in all of its glory and stink. It seems that something had just caught my attention and I simply forgot to flush when I was done vomiting. I left the damming evidence in plain sight for all to see.

After he finished urinating, he approached me and said, "I don't have any problem with your vomiting, just flush the water after you."

My immediate response was, of course, total and hysteric denial. "What are you talking about? I didn't vomit! How can you say I vomited?! It must have been someone else!" My hysteria made my heart pound so hard, I was sure it could be heard outside of the clinic.

He just looked at me and said, with utter indifference, "Okay, you didn't vomit," and continued on his way.

I was lucky it was a man who had caught me in the act, because that meant that the whole story ended as soon as it began. He went back to his business, probably forgot about it by the end of the day, and never spoke about it again. I suppose that had a woman caught me in the act, things would have developed otherwise.

On the other hand, I now know that nothing happens without a reason, and in retrospect I know that at that time point, I was not yet prepared to admit to myself that I was vomiting, as crazy as that sounds. As far as I was concerned, it was some other, unrelated entity that shoved a finger down my throat and forced the food out. This hard, embarrassing, and shameful experience in which my great secret was nearly revealed made me swear that I would never again repeat the utterly avoidable rookie mistake. This was one oath that I was able to keep.

THE TRANSITION TO BINGE EATING

Years of pushing fingers down my throat passed. The first major change occurred with my first pregnancy. There was a moment when I told myself, "Enough, give it a rest, there is no need to vomit. You can eat whatever you want and everything is okay." And indeed, for the first time in many years, I did not vomit during all of those months of pregnancy. I was pretty sure that I had put this episode behind me. I told myself, "So I've been vomiting for years. No big deal. There are far worse things in life. Here I've gotten over being beaten, and I will get over this as well. I've survived both experiences, and now I am continuing on to a new chapter in my life with a smile on my lips."

How naïve I was! I don't remember exactly how much time passed, whether a few weeks or months, from the moment I gave birth to the moment I found myself shoving my fingers down my throat again. And honestly, it doesn't really matter. I was back to my bad old habits, only this time with a much lower frequency.

I vomited every day, and sometimes several times a day in my youth, decreased the pace to once a week or two after the army, and then reduced it to once a month when I moved in with my husband-to-be. After my first child, I stabilized at once every two or three months, depending on the situation, the events, and the options I faced.

The ritual itself received a new form of expression. Since the vomiting frequency was relatively low, each occasion was cause for celebration. That is, when the opportunity to vomit came, which means when the urge matured for long enough to a level where it overtook almost my entire essence and when the environmental conditions enabled a worry-free and "fun" vomiting—that is to say no concealment, no questions, and no supervision. When that happened, an eating binge would take place that had only one purpose: to gorge on as much food as possible in order to vomit as much as possible.

I am not talking about two helpings and two desserts, but abnormal amounts that were completely irrational in composition and non-homogenous when mixed together—sour with pungent spices, sweet with salty, hot with cold, cooked with fresh. And all this with precise amounts of water between each helping to prevent taking up too much space in the stomach yet enable a smooth vomiting process later on.

At that special moment when I found myself leaning over the toilet, at that magical moment, I let it all rip out, as much as possible. Because what's the point of vomiting if you don't go all the way? You need to maximize the engorgement leading to the vomiting. Simple, right?

I Wanted to Tell Someone About My Vomiting

The first time I dared share the matter with a living, breathing individual other than myself was toward the end of the psychological therapy I had undergone during my journey for healing from asthma (as detailed in chapter 2), when I discussed the guilty feelings that had accompanied me for years over the hundreds of "let him die already" prayers I prayed as a child with my therapist. Something within me was prepared to share the great and embarrassing secret with others. It felt right to share it with my therapist, and that nothing wrong would happen if she knew as well.

At one moment, I couldn't take it anymore. I was tired of the exhausting internal dialogue going on in my mind between myself and my nagging inner voice ("Tell her!" "I can't!" "Tell her!" "I can't!"), and I suddenly found myself blurting out, in the middle of something entirely different, the words "And I also wanted to tell you that I vomit. I am a bulimic."

And then I was silent. I couldn't do or say anything. Even breathing felt like an incredible effort. I couldn't believe I had done it. I couldn't believe I had told her. I couldn't believe that I had let the words out of my mouth. It made it real, something that actually existed, and something that could no longer be hidden or repressed or buried, at least not with her. Not in that room.

I kept quiet and awaited her response. I didn't know how to answer the question "Why do you do that?" and I had no answer to "Why are you hurting yourself?" So I just kept quiet.

Fortunately, she didn't ask me anything. She just said, "Wow. I really respect the way you are sharing this. It must have been very hard to open up."

Very hard? Very hard? I couldn't keep quiet for almost half an hour. Rivers of pent-up and concealed feelings and secrets welled up and washed out of me, after all those years. In that session, we did not even discuss the vomiting itself but rather everything around it, the concealment and how hard it was to conceal.

Still, I left with a feeling that a very heavy burden had been lifted from me. I felt that I had taken a step, a small step, in facing up to my condition, but for me it was a giant leap. In the session that followed, we were already speaking specifically about eating disorders.

To the few among you who have not bumped up against the term, an eating disorder is a mental disorder that is expressed by irregular eating that is harmful to one's health, and it is considered one of the most opaque diseases of the Western world. On one side of the scale are the anorexics, who eat almost nothing and starve themselves to the brink of death and sometimes beyond. On the other are the obese (compulsive eaters) who can't stop eating and practically gorge themselves to death.

Smack in the middle are we bulimics, who "enjoy the best" of both worlds: we gorge on unhealthy amounts of food yet end up with nothing in our stomachs. So we engage in both gluttony and self-starvation. Bulimics find it easiest to conceal their condition from their environment, because most of us have non-deviant weight, which is not the case with our comrades on both ends of the scale. Either they are so thin, you can barely see them if you look at them from the side (and oversized sweatshirts can't hide their protruding bones or their condition) or they are so huge, you can see them coming from miles away. In contrast, we bulimics have a PhD in concealing our conditions.

WHY IT BEGAN

The therapist showed me that by vomiting, I was denying my body one of the three basic essentials it requires to survive and live—oxygen, water, and food. **Something within me, somewhere in my childhood and teenage years didn't really think my body deserved to live or was worthy of life.**

At that point in my life, when I was finally treating, touching, and handling the whole issue of my father and how he had impacted me, it felt very right, very logical. It also matched with the fact that **it had all started and broken out in the period of puberty that is characterized by difficult paths and crises of definition and identification of the self.**

I had never really understood why my father beat me. After all, I was a good, disciplined girl who helped around the house, did everything she was told, and worked like a mule on the family farm, which included the sheep pen and the orchard. The beatings I received were "punishment" meant for unruly, borderline-criminal children, who not only ignored boundaries but burned them down entirely.

So was I a good girl or a bad girl? This was not entirely clear to me during those formative years. On the one hand, my father glorified me, my intelligence, and my beauty every chance that he had with sentences like "You are the cherry on the cake" or "You will surely succeed in everything you do with your skills and smarts." On the other hand, he beat the stuffing out of me—for nothing! So what was I supposed to think? Was I worthy of praise or of a beating?

Another thing my therapist brought to my attention was the issue of control in my life, or more accurately, the absence of control in my life. It was decided for me that I would work in the sheep pen every day after school and every weekend, as well as in the orange orchard, whenever an extra pair of working hands was necessary. I didn't like being put to work.

School–work–school–work. No vacations and no leniency allowed, save for illness. I felt that I had no control over what was happening in my private life. Vomiting, on the other hand, was something I could control, at least up to a point. I decided when, where, and how to vomit. A twisted way of gaining control over my life, but that is what I had, and I guess that on some level that is what I needed.

Discussing my bulimia, as fascinating and liberating as it was, wasn't sufficient to get me to stop the vomiting. The psychological therapy ended, and I cured myself of my asthma, which made me very happy at the time. I shared my success with the entire world.

But at the same time, I continued concealing my bulimia

from the entire world. After all, I was a mistress of the art of concealment by this point in my life. Nonetheless, I had shared this information with another living person. Furthermore, the disease now had a formal name and an orderly diagnosis. Somehow, these two developments made dealing with the disease easier.

Even though this was a huge step for me after the years I had spent wallowing in my vomit, this was only the first, small step in recovering from the disease itself. And so it was that I continued living with the beast for a few more years, keeping it quiet in the dark dungeons of my soul.

WHAT THE SPIRITS TOLD ME

In 2013, I reached the spiritual teacher who would be my weekly companion for the next eighteen months. This time, I didn't wait for her to plumb my inner depths. As soon as she asked me why I came and what was troubling me in life, beyond a desire for spiritual development, I immediately shot back that I suffered from two mental illnesses (bulimia and bipolar disorder), an autoimmune disease (Hashimoto/hypothyroidism), and an addiction to light drugs.

When she asked which of them troubled me most, I replied immediately, "Bulimia and the drugs." Those were the two things that most impacted my daily life, and I had had quite enough of them at this point in my life. However, I lacked control in regard to them, and I needed serious help to regain that control.

I learned that the source of my emotional eating, manifested as bulimia, was not merely at the level of my personal biography, but also at the level of the biography of my eternal spirit. In other words, my spirit had incarnated on this world more than once, and these previous incarnations had developed an obsessive approach to eating, a sort of traumatic existence with a problematic mark.

To deal with my current problem in this life, it was necessary to see the incarnations that had developed this obsession. I learned that most eating disorders were caused by prejudices that the spirit had brought into the current incarnation from previous ones. I suppose that is why essential issues regarding the psychological questions about eating disorders such as "Why do anorexics not respond to the basic survival instinct and eat?" or "Why do they tend to resist therapy more than any other type of patient?" remain unanswered.

As the teacher had explained to me at our first session, "Psychology is like a lamp shining upon a painting on the wall. Here, we will examine the lamp itself, and use the hand holding the lamp."

The missing information could never be found in the mind alone. I stopped arguing and fighting with the reality I had created, either inadvertently or otherwise, and this led me to accept my condition, my illness, as a perfect state for me and for my development, which led to self-love. And that, in and of itself, as we have been told for thousands of years, led me to change and healing. **In order to get well, I had to change. There simply wasn't any "change bypass road,"**

not on the psychological level, and not on the level of the spirit.

THE SOURCES AND CAUSES OF EMOTIONAL EATING

This book is far too short to go into every detail of what I learned about my eating disorder and its psychological and spiritual sources during my journey, but I will share with you the elements that touched my heart most at the time and affected me more than the others.

Food blocks emotions. **We shove down unpleasant aspects and hard emotions like anger, frustration, insults, shame, or disappointment. We can't externalize those emotions, but we do want to eliminate them and no longer feel them, so we shove them down below into our stomach with food.**

Happy emotions don't even enter the stomach in the first place; at most they descend to our heart, pass through our throat, and are there externalized. We share the happiness, the joy, the excitement. Those are pleasant emotions, easy and light, and they cannot be condensed.

In the case of anger or any other difficult emotion that we judge as negative, the jaws are immediately activated, since chewing contributes to the dimming and the release of that anger or another hard emotion.

When I felt off, confused, or inadequate during childhood, that thought whose essence was "something is wrong with me" was shoved into my body. **Any other undesirable**

thoughts that we shunt aside, try to ignore, forget, or suppress don't really leave or disappear, but enter our body, which is one of the main causes for diseases.

Whenever I feel even the slightest pain, I know now that what I must ask straightaway is "What is the thought I just tried to avoid or suppress?" I know now that distasteful thoughts must not be shoved into the dark dungeon. Instead, I express gratitude for them until they dissipate.

Even if I am in the middle of a session of emotional eating, I know I must give thanks, since in a state of thankfulness, it is not possible to be in the past or the future but only in the here and now. Nor does it really matter who you give thanks to—just be in the moment, be in it completely, and the thought will dissipate on its own. I tried this approach several times and was surprised to see that it worked.

One of the more significant surprises on this journey, which also formed a turning point in my attitude toward the disease, was the knowledge that by vomiting, I was also expelling unwanted energy. The food was mixing in with the negative energy, annexing the frustration, sadness, helplessness, and mostly the great fear that I felt, and then I vomited them all out together, outside of me.

I had to learn to respect what I had gone through, not blame myself for the tendency to vomit, and even forgive myself for condemning myself for the vomiting. The vomiting episodes were not unalloyed evil, they also contained goodness and even a measure of relief.

CASE STUDY

One evening, my husband and my older children went to a new movie I really wanted to see, but we couldn't find a babysitter so I had to stay with the baby at home. The second the car doors slammed shut, I immediately approached the refrigerator and started gorging myself. There was no thought involved, just pure auto-pilot. A few days later I finally understood what had kindled that automatic response.

As soon as my husband and older children had left the house, I began feeling intense pangs of jealousy. "I am jealous they are going to the film and that I am stuck at home," a feeling that I judged as being unworthy and inappropriate. This thought was accompanied by repression of those emotions, with the thought "There is something wrong with me for feeling anger and jealousy," and from there, the route to self-punishment and gorging was extremely short because **the food both suppressed these emotions and was a form of punishment for them.**

This is an extremely rapid process that occurs within less than a second: a negative thought > negative self-judgment (from childhood conditioning) > suppression of the emotion by emotional eating. So simple, but so painful and sad.

To summarize, I will share that we also carried out a "transformational regression" session, which is a return to a previous incarnation in order to repair that incarnation and disable past frequencies from affecting us, in my case emotional eating frequencies. The experience in which this prior incarnation is viewed is not a mere fact-finding tour de force to arrive at the proper solution; it is, since everything within it happens simultaneously, the solution itself.

I admit that to this day, I am unable to comprehend the "making whole that occurs simultaneously in all dimensions" business with my three-dimensional human brain, but it felt right to do this even without understanding it, and I am happier for it. In that session, I could see how I had used food to control other people in a previous incarnation. I asked forgiveness from the spirits that had been caught up in the harmful conduct of my prior incarnation, and it led me to understand, at a level far beyond the rational and conscious, why I had created an existence in which food controlled me. A lesson in self-control on the food front.

Some spirits inflict lessons of self-control on the erotic front (sex addicts), the economic front (gamblers, kleptomaniacs), or the work front (workaholics). There are plenty of lessons available, and each and every one of us has a lesson we selected for ourselves with the goal of assuming self-control, since it is the only thing that enables us to choose the desirable, pleasant, and longed-for experiences in life.

THE LAST TIME

I knew, deep within, that one day it would all disappear, and so it happened. Toward the end of my studies with my spiritual mentor, around September 2014, I was busy one evening with overeating, a foolish gluttony, and I heard an inner voice tell me, "This is it. You are not throwing up anymore. We're done with it. You will have to face up to the consequences of this gorging. Today you are going to sleep with a swollen stomach and that's it."

That is when I knew, just knew, that I was really done with shoving fingers down my throat. The temptation was great at that point because my stomach was already hurting and it is no fun, no fun at all, to go to sleep with a swollen stomach. But for the first time in my life, I was able to control it and went to sleep with that swollen belly from a place of self-compassion, clapping virtual hands at my accomplishment.

That's it, I am no longer throwing up. I still had to deal with emotional eating, and it took me almost a year from the moment I stopped vomiting to reach a point where I felt I had emotional eating under control. It was not simple for me that year, not in the least, since I was making a big effort to maintain correct and healthy nutrition, yet I suddenly found myself opening a box of chocolate spread or eating various other sweet nonsense. The amounts were truly minute and minor, but I could sense that they were anything but cute little "I want something sweet right now" whims. Oh no. They were coming from far deeper and darker places.

Still, at this stage in my life, I knew that there was no point in fighting this situation or getting bummed out by it. There was nothing to do but accept it and accept myself along with it.

Then one day, it was over. One day, I woke up to the knowledge that weeks had gone by without an emotional eating attack. I had won back self-control. Today, I can say that my nutrition is a way of showing myself, through my stomach and intestines, that I really love myself. I can certainly allow myself an "I feel like something sweet" whim here and there. It is all just a matter of dosage.

SUMMARY

To summarize, what did bulimia teach me about myself?

- The extent to which I hated and didn't really accept myself and that my body was worthy of life and love.
- I had to give harsh emotions legitimacy and expression, and not suppress or punish myself.
- I took back control of my life, on the emotional, mental, and behavioral levels.

CHAPTER 7
ADDICTION TO LIGHT DRUGS (CANNABIS)

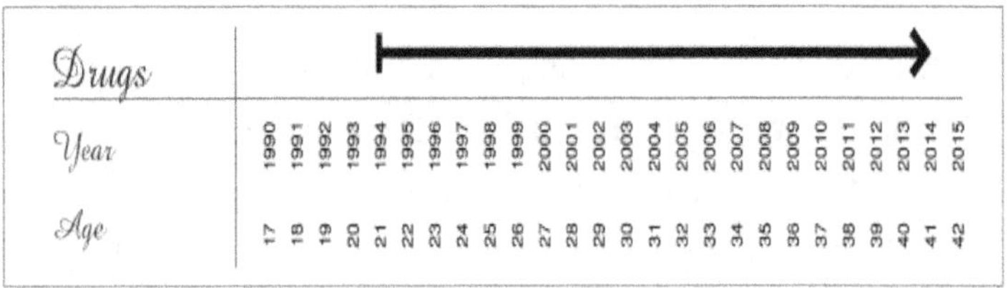

I smoked my first joint when I was twenty. My first experience with dimming out reality was extremely powerful, and found a very receptive and febrile mind. I certainly had a deep, subconscious need to escape reality as it was, to flee the turbulent and suppressed emotions that filled the dank dungeon of my soul.

As a professional pothead in good standing, I prayed to get my hands on good weed that would let me recapture this experience, to feel those sensations just as powerfully as the first time, and to fly as high as I had that first time, including mad laughter. I wish even ten percent of the many, many joints I smoked in my life were like that first one. The truth, unfortunately, was light-years away.

I limited my joint-smoking sessions to evenings for a decade. And when I say evenings, I mean each and every evening and at least five joints an evening, because I couldn't function professionally when I was high. Given the field I was in (advertising), this is quite surprising, since half of the workers in the field, particularly in the Copyright and Art Design departments, smoked light drugs throughout the day, and in some firms, they didn't even bother going outside to do so. They say it improves their creativity, and who can argue with results?

As for myself, a single experimental joint in the middle of the work day was enough to make clear to me that if I wanted to remain employed I had to confine my joint sessions to the evening. At the time, I was an account executive in an advertising firm.

One day, a copywriter and I left the studio where we had been recording radio commercials. He took out the "after-recording joint" and offered to share. I was in a good mood since everything was coming along properly and, for a change, there were no fires for me to put out in the office. It was late in the afternoon and a tone of "maybe I'll leave for home early today when there is still daylight" was in the air, so I agreed.

We had a very pleasant smoke, ordered a cab, and returned to the office. When I answered a call from one of my clients, I realized that I was unable to focus on the conversation, unable to understand what she was talking about, couldn't follow her. I must have muttered something unclear, because she suddenly stopped and asked me, "Tell me, are you all right?"

When I denied anything was wrong, she told me that I didn't sound too good and asked whether I was feeling well. I leapt at the opportunity and immediately told her that I had a headache and that I had been suffering from dizziness over the past hour. She suggested I go home, and I gratefully agreed.

I realized that my brain was unable to process information rapidly in the focused, system-wide, and multilevel manner my job required. After this experience, I learned my lesson, and to the end of my days as an employee, I never again got high in the middle of a work day.

A Woman With a Box

Not smoking in the daytime on weekdays did not prevent me from smoking on the weekend from the moment I got up in the morning to the moment I passed out at night, and did not prevent me from arriving at every social event with "the box." This sweet and beloved magic box was my constant companion wherever I went. There was no chance that I would arrive at any social event without my box.

In my early years, I was still dependent on my veteran pothead friends who would bring their boxes, the boon companions of any self-respecting pothead. After I had smoked a joint or two that I had rolled up at home and brought over in a cigarette box, I would sit and wait for that well-known box of surprises to emerge from one of the bags.

Every pothead knows the feeling of anticipation for a pot buddy's box.

Everyone around me smoked; there were almost no non-smokers in the group. But only a few had "magic boxes," because most of them smoked the material of the "box people." The longer one smokes pot, you see, the higher the dosage of active ingredient in the joint has to be in order to have an effect, since the old dosage simply doesn't affect the smokers as much anymore. (In professional jargon, it's called "developing tolerance.")

As the years passed and I gained experience, I too became a woman with a box. I even took the box with me when I flew abroad. Of course, the box was empty in the airport—I wasn't quite that devoid of my senses—but I would pad my bra with a small amount. Just one or two fixes to make sure I was never without. It never took me more than a few hours to find the local supplier (you can always find one), but I didn't ever want to be stuck without my fix.

As far as I was concerned, it was pure agony not to be high during a vacation. Hell, it was agony not to be high every free moment of each day, but particularly so on vacations, which is why almost all of our vacations were in Egypt's Sinai Peninsula. Sinai was a classic pothead vacation in which one could spend all day on the beach, never more than a meter away from the lean-to we slept in. There was no need to move, and there is nothing a pothead likes better than "no need to move."

The kids could horse around to their great enjoyment, and there weren't even any electronic screens to distract them (or the adults) from the sea, sand, and wind. Just a whole week of nothing to do but lie on your back and flip over occasionally, and go to a restaurant to eat once in a while.

A "win-win" situation as it's called in the business world, which made feeling good and being open about my addiction much easier. I never hid this particular illness; on the contrary, I openly admitted for years that I was addicted to light drugs. I had no problem with this addiction. I even liked it—or thought I did. It was part of me, I could not imagine my life without it, and I didn't really want to, because it brought me great joy. I loved being a smoker, both of cigarettes and joints.

In retrospect, I think the reason I didn't hide the fact that I was addicted to light drugs, either from myself or others, was related to the fact that I did hide so many other things for so many years that I viewed as truly horrible. That was not, as I viewed the world, the case with my joints. I viewed my bulimia and bipolar disorder as far more horrible so I hid them accordingly. My friends, in contrast, always insisted I was exaggerating with my description of myself as an addict, and most refused to label themselves as such.

WHO'S THE BOSS?

According to the dictionary, addiction is a "situation of psychological and/or physical dependence on a substance or activity, which is characterized by compulsive behavior meant to achieve that stimulus which continues even when it leads to negative consequences."

In other words, you are addicted when your addiction is managing you. You are addicted when you are not the one running the show. You are addicted when the narcotic substance is dictating where you go (most likely wherever you can find drugs), who to see (most likely whoever has drugs), when to see them (most likely when they have drugs and you don't), and when to leave (most likely when the drugs are all gone). A surefire way to test whether you are an addict is to consider your behavior during times of shortage, when the police shut down a border crossing that the drug smugglers use.

What do you do when you, your supplier, and your close friends, even those with a cancer-patient relative with a medical prescription, are all out? You find yourself picking up the phone and calling people whose company you don't care for and who you haven't even talked to over the past year, just on the off chance that you might be surprised and get a small chunk of hashish or even the raw cannabis plant.

This neediness takes over your entire essence, and it makes you do things you wouldn't do in any other situation. Every pothead has occasionally found himself driving to the other side of town, even at midnight, just to "borrow" a small fix to tide him through the night.

Sounds terrible, doesn't it? It sounds like the behavior of heroin mainliners who can't live for a single moment without their fix, right? But hey, ask the potheads and nicotine smokers what happens when their joints are all gone without any early preparation? What happens when they want to smoke but there is no box in the house or anyone else smoking next to them? How many drawers in the house do they turn inside out? How many nicotine crumbs do they gather from these drawers to try to find a sufficient amount to tide them over until morning? How many of them will bang on the doors of smoking neighbors or leave in the middle of the night to get some cigarettes from the nearest gas station or 24/7 kiosk, no matter how bad the weather is?

As far as I was concerned, this behavior, which was my behavior as well, met the basic criteria for an addiction. It didn't really matter to me whether my friends agreed with this definition or didn't. How they chose to define their condition was their choice. As far as I was concerned, I viewed myself as an addict. But I enjoyed it, in spite of the technical difficulties this addiction posed for me.

In 2010, I ended the wage-worker chapter of my life, and I moved on to be independently employed. On the practical level, I worked from home, and I pretty much controlled my own time. I didn't always know what to do with all of my free time, and I found myself spending many hours alone with myself, which of course slowly led to a growing need to escape myself every once in a while, because I didn't know what the hell to do with all of this alone time.

I found myself puffing at a joint in the early afternoon and sneaking a noon puff every few days. I made sure I finished the tasks requiring human interaction as soon as possible, including photography for the program I presented on, and I would seat myself with my box and roll up my sweet noon joint.

In 2011, I stopped smoking nicotine cigarettes during a pivotal eight-day juice fast, which meant I automatically transitioned to smoking even more joints as compensation. I chose to view it as a whole: I used to smoke both cigarettes and pot, but now I was pot-exclusive. I had reduced my nicotine intake, which was the truly addictive trash, and that was good enough for me.

As the years passed, the timing of the first puff came earlier and earlier, and in the summer of 2013, when my fourth child was born and I found myself awake at inhumane hours like 5:30 a.m., I broke all self-imposed limitations and rolled up an early (very early) morning joint.

A WATERSHED MOMENT

At this point, my initial pleasure with the drug high had been replaced with fatigue. Ten minutes after smoking a joint, if I wasn't at the keyboard working or writing, all I wanted to do was sleep…bad, which led me to do as little as possible. All of the things I wanted to initiate, promote, or get done kept on getting postponed to another opportunity or to the pothead classic "tomorrow morning."

I consoled myself by telling myself that I had always known what to do, I functioned very well with drugs, I had worked full-time with the drugs, I had earned a university degree with the drugs, I had changed careers with the drugs, I had raised wonderful kids with the drugs, and I had slowly evolved to new places with the drugs.

The watershed moment in regard to my addiction came one ordinary afternoon sometime in 2011, when I was smoking a joint in the garden and an inner voice told me, "You no longer need drugs. They have done their part. Now you are simply addicted to them."

My entire essence knew that this insight was completely on the mark. Some insights in life just make themselves apparent, and we all experience special moments like this. That is the moment when, for the first time in my smoke-screened life as an adult, a desire was born to stop smoking drugs. I had never before wanted to stop smoking drugs or fought an inner need to stop smoking, because no such need existed. This need was suddenly born in a single watershed moment and created, *ex nihilo*, a desire to wean myself from the dependence on drugs.

That was how I initiated my road of independence from drugs, a road that took me three years to walk. These three years had quite a few drug-free intermissions, some of them successfully lasting several months. They also had quite a few exhausting and painful falls off the wagon and many, many bouts of self-flagellation:

Why am I doing this to myself?

I'm sick of myself.

Why do I smoke?

I hate drugs.

I'll never be able to stop—it's stronger than me.

I am such a fuck-up.

And other such depressing morsels.

My desire to put an end to my drug habit led me to examine the causes of my addiction and consider what petri dish they had settled on. Dealing with harsh emotions and anxieties, including an insane work pressure in the advertising field, combined with an inability to deal with too many negative emotions and stress (both in my work environment and from childhood), led me to use addictive substances as a means to relieve those emotional-mental anxieties and as a source of immediate relief. That same pleasant, softening, dimming sensation led to me to puff on the joint again and again, all the way to addiction and to long-term dependence.

That's all well and good, but these reflections did not advance me toward freedom from addiction. Theoretical knowledge about the psychological-behavioral sources of my addiction did not promote application in the field that would enable withdrawal. Even the fact that a supply crisis led to a rise in the cost my monthly drug supplies by over a thousand dollars a month did not stop me from smoking all day long.

When you smoke drugs—and it really doesn't matter whether they are heavy or light drugs—you want to get to a place where none of that bothers you, a place where you can escape your problems, large or small, a place where you can see things from a slightly different perspective. And it works...for a second and a half to an hour and a half (depending on the drug).

The problem is that you land back in reality, but nothing changes there because the drugs are merely an attempt to escape, and you can't really escape. You can't escape the reality, and you can't escape all the inner demons dwelling in the dungeon down below, some of them for many years, lurking in wait for us until the right moment arrives for them to pounce. One of the fears that stalks those who desire to end their addiction is the fear of what lies in wait. What sleeping hounds will awaken when the narcotic haze wears off? This fear is identical to the fear of listening to our wounded and bleeding soul. Who knows what story it might tell me about myself? Perhaps I won't like the story. Maybe I won't be able to live with it. Maybe it will make me hate myself even more than I already do. This fear can paralyze you for years.

CAREFULLY PRESELECTED SITUATIONS

In the spring of 2013, I reached my spiritual teacher from whom I received information by channeling the sources of my addiction both on the level of my soul (the product of my biography in this existence) and on the spiritual plane (the level that is the product of my spirit's existence in all of its incarnations).

On the one hand, this stressed me out. If my eternal spirit had been unable to take care of its business and deal with its hang-ups, then how could I, the temporal body "from dust thou hast come and to dust thou shalt return", survive? It felt to me that there was no chance for success and that I would always run internal dialogues and arguments such as this:

"I am sick of smoking, it isn't good for me."

"Smoke. Come on, take a puff. It will do you good and relieve your stress."

"Damn, why did I smoke? Now I don't feel like doing anything, and I also have the munchies."

"Well, you deserve it."

This pressure resulted in negative reactions, such as periods of greater smoking. My baggage of pain, which was the sum of all negative energies accumulated by my spirit throughout its many lives, was working overtime.

On the other hand, I learned that these situations were carefully selected so that I would have the opportunity to choose to overcome them, and thereby repair, both on the level of my temporal soul and on the level of the eternal spirit, which mostly existed on a higher dimension than our three-dimensional-linear universe. I received a great deal of encouragement not to fight the addiction, because whatever you resist is empowered by that resistance.

I also received a lot of encouragement to continue to shine light on the shadowed places and to believe that the day would come when I would no longer need drugs—the day I could choose not to smoke. I was promised unambiguously that day would come.

"Be certain that the day will come when you are completely indifferent to the sight of a joint lying next to you, just as you are already indifferent to the sight of a cigarette box on the table."

Until that day arrived, I had to let go of my war on drugs and end my self-flagellation, and even enjoy my joints, so long as they served me on some level.

I learned to accept myself as I was, and I could do that only after I learned not to fight reality but to accept it, because the reality I experienced and created was exactly right for me. It was exactly what my spirit needed and was linked to my destiny on Earth and the fulfillment of my purpose on it. If I took a puff on a joint after an intermission of three months, that was exactly the way it was supposed to be.

Wow, this was a major change in perception. A crazy transition from the concept of "Life is happening to me and I have no control over it" to "I am creating whatever is happening to me in life for my own supernal good." I remember that on the first Saturday I abstained from puffing on a joint, I asked myself repeatedly, "All right, so what do I do with all of this unalloyed and undimmed reality?"

Living reality with clarity, without any dimming whatsoever to shield me from its harsh angles and sharp corners, was certainly something that took time to get used to. I could no longer run anywhere. Reality and life hit me with all their power and, at first, I simply couldn't contain it. I was blinded by the light, so I went back to puffing on my joints in order to dim reality and shade down the light. I stopped, repeated, was bummed out, stopped, returned, and was bummed out so many times in those years, but nonetheless accepted the fact that I needed my joints, and smoked with almost no guilty feelings.

I knew that it would pass at the best time for me, even if I couldn't see it at that moment. I believed that it was possible for anyone to free himself from any addiction, but I had to replace the addiction with something else, something positive and empowering. I waited, most of the time rather patiently, for this positive replacement to arrive.

Smelling the End

In September 2014, I ended studies with my spiritual teacher, since I had decided to embark on my own way without her support. Something within me told me that I had to apply all of the tools and knowledge I received on my own and consult with myself about the way to proceed. That the answers would come, as the immortal cliché said.

I was still smoking the occasional joint, but my relationship with the addiction was in a totally different place than four years before. I won't exaggerate by saying that this was a positive place, but it certainly wasn't the same combative place but rather, an accepting and containing place.

At that exact same time, a friend asked me to go to a meeting on his behalf to get an impression of what "One Brain" was all about. It was an extremely smart treatment method based on kinesiology, a direct conversation with the subconscious via muscle response to queries. The body never lies, and it reveals to a therapist, fairly quickly, where the emotional blocks inhibiting or paining the patient are hidden, usually since their childhood. A "bullshit bypass road."

I fell in love with the system and underwent a number of sessions. Within the framework of those treatments, I discovered, among other things, that deep within me existed a belief that I was not worthy of this life and that life itself provided proof of this fact. In parallel, life had led me to a study class called "bio-orgonomy."

In this class, I was granted the opportunity of seeing how miracles—large and small, simple and complex—occurred. The bio-orgonomy method is a diagnosis and treatment method based on the assumption that everybody has an energy field, and that a sick individual is missing energy in an organ, limb, or the entire body. The bio-orgonomy treatment rehabilitated its energetic state, restoring its self-healing potential, and enabled recovery.

The belief that miracles do indeed occur under specific and very precise conditions, in accordance to a mysterious master plan, slowly formed within me. Toward the end of the course, I began parallel "multisensory meditation" studies, and in their framework, I learned how to tap into my higher self on a daily basis.

On the last day of my bio-orgonomy studies, two weeks before I had completed my drug withdrawal, a fellow studying with me approached suddenly and passed along the following message: "You know, every person has a sort of a ring at the end of his aura, at the top of his head. When you smoke drugs, you are allowing foreign entities and energies to enter your aura through this ring. If you don't do drugs, they will no longer be able to enter." He added that he usually didn't do this, asked for forgiveness if his words had offended me because that was not his intention, and carried on with his business.

His words did not fall on deaf ears. I knew that this

message was intended for me. I shared it with another student, who had discovered during the studies that she had both healing abilities beyond the comprehension of the human brain and a type of "x-ray vision" that was capable of seeing things that could not be explained.

This friend heard my words, saw what she saw, and told me, "It is clear that you will succeed in overcoming your addiction, because this is only the beginning of your way. You will reach far."

The entire period when I learned to do and heal with energetic work and even practiced it repeatedly, I heard an inner voice telling me that if I wished to reach a maximum ability and even miracles, as I had seen with others, I would have to let go of the drugs. And yet, all of these things were not enough to get me to let go of drugs in practice.

THE POWER OF PRAYER

Two weeks after the messages from my fellow students and a month after the "one mind" treatment session came an evening when I returned to puffing on joints after a few good days I had stayed on the wagon. It made me feel terrible both physically and emotionally. The frustration and despair were so great that I found myself raising my eyes to the ceiling and praying to God.

"Please, please, please," I begged him, for the first time in my life. "Please help me help myself. I can't do it alone. Please, please help me." I was weeping in despair, and then

I went to bed.

When I woke up in the morning, I knew at once that my prayer had been answered. I knew that I would never smoke cannabis again. Ever. I just had this absolute knowledge that God had heard me and had accepted my plea. That is the simplest way to describe what happened.

Aside from the help of the big boss in Heaven, which cannot be discounted, the right moment had arrived. The powerful desire I felt to get in touch with my source of strength overcame my desire to be high and the addiction itself. The addiction to something external ended as soon as I found my sought-after alternative: the addiction to something internal, the power within myself.

On December 2014, at the age of forty-one, after twenty-one years, the need and desire to flee from myself disappeared and never returned. As was promised to me almost a year earlier by the sentient entities that communicated with me through my spiritual teacher, the day came when I found myself indifferent to the sight of a joint, and even indifferent to the sight of people around me smoking joints.

From the day I stopped smoking to the time these pages were published, I have attended dozens of parties and social functions where my old friends still puffed away like there was no tomorrow. I don't mind. In every past attempt to stop smoking drugs, I was always jealous of the smokers. I felt they were having fun while I was miserable.

Those days are now behind me. Not only am I not jealous, I am incredibly happy that I am no longer in that place. I am out of the trap. I am back in control. I am done with running away from reality. I am connected to my inner strength.

SUMMARY

What did my addiction to drugs teach me about myself?

- I was running from myself, as well as from my past. I was incapable of living with myself.
- I was high and drugging out the demons within, because I was afraid that the ugly truth would get me to hate myself more than I already did.
- Smoking pot was the only way I could overcome so many hard feelings, stress, and pressure (from childhood and work).
- I learned how to grow addicted to myself and my inner strength.

CHAPTER 8
HYPOTHYROIDISM ROUND 2

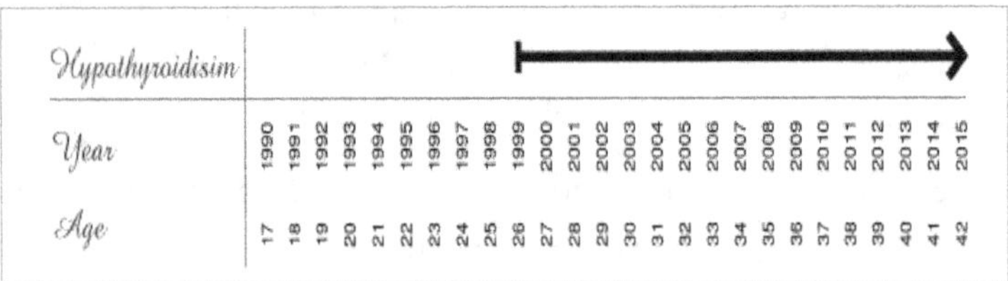

On March 21, 2015, at 1:01 in the morning, something woke me from a deep sleep, a phrase appearing in my mind: "Disease is the language of the soul." I opened my laptop, which lay at the foot of my bed, saw the time, and felt a strong inkling that I was embarking on a new path. I typed in the phrase I had woken up with: Disease is the language of the soul.

Over the next four hours, I entered a frenzy of writing and finished the first two pages of a book. Can I honestly say that I knew what I was writing? Not really. Was it really me who wrote the first two chapters of the book? I'm not too sure about that either. In any event, that is how this book came to be written.

At that point in time, I was proud of all of my achievements.

I was healthy, happy, and without pills, just the way I wanted. My satisfaction was overshadowed by the fact that I couldn't restore my thyroid gland to full functionality in spite of my many efforts, but I understood that some things were simply out of my hands. I did what I could, and believed, and knew that when the right day arrived, my TSH blood counts would be sound and my thyroid gland would function properly.

On May 13, 2015, my family physician, for the first time in our fifteen years together, took initiative and asked to examine my routine blood assays for the presence of antibodies to the enzyme thyroid peroxidase, which has a critical role in the production of thyroid gland hormones. These are autoimmune antibodies formed by the immune system when it malfunctions, for reasons unclear to medical science, targeting elements of the body itself rather than external invasive factors, leading the antibodies to act against the cells of the body and bring about the destruction of its tissues and disruption of the function of the thyroid gland.

Two aberrant findings stuck out of that assay: the TSH levels had leapt to 42.56, and the antibodies, whose normal range was 0–35, were measured at 702!

The doctor was delighted to confirm what he had suspected and searched for, and joy was not exactly his normal baseline state. He explained to me in simple terms what these findings meant.

"See," he told me, all excited, pointing at the screen, "I found out why your thyroid gland has not been functioning over all these years. It's your antibodies—they are attacking it."

"Hold on," I snapped. "If this parameter is so basic, how can this be the first time someone bothered to think to perform this test?" A feeling of déjà vu began to overwhelm me. Could history be repeating itself? "Why, in all of the sixteen years in which my blood tests revealed a distinct diagnosis of hypothyroidism, didn't any doctor stop to check out these antibodies in a simple blood assay?" I asked him. "Why didn't anybody check for these antibodies like you have, if they are the culprits assailing the thyroid gland?"

I just couldn't believe that once again no one had noticed. The doctor was so excited with the results that he just told me that the important thing was that the cause of my troubles had been identified.

HERE WE GO AGAIN

That was the opening salvo of the first battle in this round with hypothyroidism. I felt much as I had in 2007, when the hypothyroidism had been formally diagnosed, but this time I was much more knowledgeable and experienced from many, many failed attempts to get well.

A month later, I arrived for the appointment I had set up with the homeopath physician who had accompanied me through my fourth pregnancy. I presented him with the new data and asked him for an action plan. That was when I felt the motivation to do whatever was necessary to cure my thyroid gland. I left with a long and detailed chart of everything I had to do, not only to return my thyroid gland to balance, but also to repair all of my body's systems. My pH level was far too acidic, and I had a severe shortage of magnesium and iron and all sorts of other deficiencies, which led him to laugh and say he could not understand how I could function under these conditions and even arrive at the office with a smile.

My body, the masterwork machine always striving to balance and programmed accordingly, had learned to balance itself even under conditions of deficiency. One thing compensated for another, and a shortage in a given mineral was compensated by robbing Peter to pay Paul—anything to keep it balanced. That was how I was able to bear three years of deficiencies in hormones critical to the body.

And not only had I not experienced most of the side effects typical of this hypothyroidism, I sometimes experienced an opposite effect. For example, hypothyroidism is generally typified by severe fatigue or weakness, whereas I was filled with energy and floated along most of the days as if I were a love-struck girl of sixteen. I had no constipation, no depression, no skin dryness, no disruption of my monthly period, and no weight gain, in spite of my extremely low metabolism. I did experience significant hair loss, but almost any woman who has gone through several pregnancies can say the same, that we have long lost our thick manes of hair.

The chart I left the doctor with included many food additives, which I immediately ordered from abroad (I received a referral to specific products from specific companies). They cost me quite a bit of money, and were supposed to maintain my entire body, not merely my thyroid gland, in a true and holistic balance that would also be reflected in my blood tests.

No more balancing acts supported by no more than my willpower and desire to be balanced and well, but a scientifically based balance. I entered into a strict nutritional regime yet again, which included the additives and various other substances I had to ingest. Some of them, like the iodine and the baking soda, outright repulsive. The regime included a close follow-up and daily measurement of the pH levels in my urine, and particular strict attention to nutrition, which at this stage of my life was already composed almost entirely from natural substances (vegetables, fruit, legumes, grains, eggs, nuts, and small quantities of meat).

The regime also included daily energetic work on meditation itself, during which I imagined the antibodies leaving my thyroid gland in peace and allowing it to return to life. I could literally see the color "return to its cheeks" and take flight like a butterfly (the shape of the thyroid gland resembles a butterfly), and return to pulse in its proper place in my neck.

Furthermore, I thanked my damaged organs and systems for teaching me a valuable lesson about wellness and health. I already knew that life was so precise, so much not a function of chance—that everything taking place was happening for my own betterment, but that this would rarely go hand in hand with my immediate benefit. I could do nothing but accept reality as it was and be thankful for the challenge I received, for it contained, in spite of the many obstacles and disappointments along the way, my great opportunity.

The strict regimen that began in June was partially interrupted in August due to a family trip abroad. I took my bag of additives along with me and I was careful to inject all of them, including the most repulsive. I was extra careful to observe my nutritional instructions; I had to keep providing my body with what it needed. However, the trip did not leave any time or space for meditation, the energetic work, or writing the book. In the beginning of September, with the long-awaited return of the children to kindergarten and school, I returned to partial energetic work and to thankfulness.

On October 6, I took a blood test to see the results of this strict regimen. I was very excited, but I was no longer hopeful or praying for a good result. I knew that whatever the test would show was the exact result I needed. The results came in two days later, on October 8, 2015.

Why is that date important? Because on that day, I visited a special conference of Kryon in Israel. Kryon is a magnetic entity, literally from out of this world, that transmits its information to humanity through a kindly American engineer by the name of Lee Carol. This information is intended to aid humanity in evolving to the next level of consciousness.

During the conference, two direct channelings were performed. (For those who have no idea what "channeling" is, I will only say that this engineer sat on the stage and the entity spoke through him to transmit its message. You can feel in your heart whether it is real or not. There will always be doubters, and it's fine to be in doubt).

The first channeling was performed during the lunch

break. It was about how God was within each and every one of us and that all we needed to do was open our hearts to Him. He spoke of how the God of Israel was the God of all of humanity and always had been. He spoke about how, in the past, humanity had moved from the commandment of law (the Ten Commandments) to the commandment of love, and we were now slowly moving to the commandment of compassion.

He spoke of how humanity's relationship with the world of spirit or God was very different after a thousand years, for mankind was evolving spiritually and was now receiving messages directly.

Oh My God!

Why am I going on and on about something that sounds more than a little bizarre, whose source is an amorphic magnetic entity? And what does all this have to do with me getting well? I'm dwelling on this because everything is connected; that's how this world works. Unfortunately, when you disregard this essential fact, you suffer. Well, you suffer more.

So let's get back to this lunch break at the Kryon conference, which I attended with a pounding heart and the feeling that God had spoken to me directly. Throughout the twenty-minute channeling, I felt God in my heart. It is hard to explain what this means on a rational level, because this is something that you experience on many levels: physiological, emotional, and spiritual. I felt that I already knew these things, that I was simply recalling them, and that inner voice that had accompanied me throughout this long path was screaming at me that I would no longer be the same person.

Dizzy with the experience, my sister (who had attended the conference with me) and I were famished. (God or no God, when the stomach is rumbling you've got to eat.) We walked toward the place where we wanted to eat lunch, and I received an email from the hospital that the final blood test results for my thyroid gland had come in.

I accessed the site, clicked on the results tab, and saw that my TSH levels had leapt to 52. Just like that—a good, round figure without any decimal point or fractions. I blurted out, "Oh my God!" Even though I had made a point of not having any expectations or hopes, this was a result I really wasn't expecting.

My sister glanced at the result and said immediately, "Well, as you taught me, it's always darkest before the dawn, right?" The moment I heard that, I knew that I had heard exactly what I needed to hear, and knew that I didn't know how to deal with that at that moment and had to let go. I chose not to do anything until I knew what I had to do, if I even had to do anything.

So we ordered lunch and returned to the conference. I sent the doctor the results of the blood tests by email and asked him, "What do you think God is trying to tell me with this?" After all, it simply made no sense that after all of this supplement regime, all of my efforts on all fronts and channels, and the significant improvement in my physiological parameters, my thyroid gland hormone levels showed such a severe deterioration. That was simply insane.

The unknown was greater than the known to both myself and my physician, and we couldn't make sense of it. He sent me back an email with a single word: "Damn." I loved him for this answer, I loved the humanity in this honesty. He didn't know how to process these results either, and he chose not to conceal his difficulties from me. It was very human, and completely different from how other doctors had responded to mistakes over the years, because they had been trained to conceal empathy and emotions in order to be better physicians.

He asked me to stop all of the nutritional supplements and everything else, and then to take another blood test to assess the effect of halting everything. His request to halt the treatment matched my inner feeling that I had to let go at this point, but it was not an easy place to be in. I still believed I would make it, I still believed I would cure my thyroid gland, but believing something that contradicted observable reality was a true trial of faith.

A War Between the Mind and the Heart

I knew that my faith was on the line here. My own binding of Isaac. That night, I dialed up God. I just sat on the bed and asked him to give me the strength to withstand this trial. I asked him the sixty-four-thousand-dollar question: "Why? Why is all this happening?"

I got an answer. "Carry on. Things will work out." This sentence that showed up in my mind, supposedly as just another thought, one of the myriad thoughts running through my skull on a daily basis, was accompanied by a comforting feeling in the heart that all was well. I found myself in tears, seemingly for no good reason, felt the good in my heart, and a few seconds later, the mind kicked in. Of course. It always has something to say and that's fine with me. That's its job and it is simply performing it. My brain was telling me that there was no way that I could cure my thyroid gland from the abysmal condition it had reached. There was simply no way.

I was caught, once again, in a war between my mind and heart. An ancient war between what my heart felt and what my mind knew. The message I got was not exactly "Take off your sandals, for the place where you are standing is holy ground" but was instead "Well, you haven't introduced anything new to me, God."

But the sensation in my heart was new and I could feel it. I had learned throughout my life that there was no reasoning with emotions because when you feel something, you feel it, and you know that you feel it, even if you later suppress, bury, or deny it. I could feel God in my heart. So in order to make peace between my quarrelsome brain and heart, I asked God to give me the strength to carry on and give me a sign that everything was all right. I needed it.

During the month of the break in my treatment, the only thing I did was a simple series of exercises daily, an ancient and fun set known as the Five Tibetan Rites. These are five dreadfully simple physical exercises, each of which needs to be repeated twenty-one times. Its source is in the Tibetan monasteries, and it was brought to the West in the beginning of the twentieth century by a retired British officer, who had himself learned it from Tibetan lamas in a monastery in the Himalaya Mountains.

This daily exercise improves physical strength and flexibility and simultaneously improves one's clarity of thought. In parallel, the exercises themselves work on and with the energetic network in our body, including the energy nodes known as chakras. A few years earlier, I was already exercising with this series for a period of time after reading that the body of the officer who had introduced this series had grown younger with time. The exercises slowed his aging process, and at the age of seventy, he looked no older than forty-five.

At the time, I jumped at the bargain and practiced the exercises for two months. It was really fun, because it takes ten to eleven minutes, a minimal investment of time and effort, but I couldn't really see any results (I'm still not clear on what exactly I was expecting to happen in two months), and I abandoned the exercises.

Why did I return to those exercises even though I said I would do nothing in regard to the thyroid gland during that month? Because my sister, the one who had joined me in the Kryon conference, called me up one day and told me that she was inspired to return to exercising the Five Tibetans. I was infected with her inspiration at that moment. Some things bypass reason. They take you over and don't let go, and so it was with the Tibetan exercises.

Some Help from the Angels

On November 8, exactly one month after the Kryon convention where I discovered the severe deterioration in the condition of my thyroid gland, I did something active. One day, a friend arrived at my home without early warning and told me how a certain treatment had cured her knees and prevented her from undergoing a planned operation at the last moment. I needed to do no more than pick up the phone and set up an appointment for myself. After all, why should she benefit and not me? Why not give it a try? It certainly couldn't hurt.

This is a treatment that lasted an hour with a special channeler who, in addition to receiving information from external entities, like any self-respecting channeler, also served as a channel or pipeline through which healing passes on several levels—physical, mental, emotional, and energetic—all according to the specific needs of that person at that time. The healing comes from entities and angels who do not wear physical forms or even manifest on our dimension, who desire to help you and advance you one more step toward realizing your vision, destination, and spiritual purpose.

In addition, I received reinforcement so that I could tell everyone that we do indeed create our own reality, that we create our own diseases, and that there is significance as to the type of disease and its location. Most importantly, I was meant to pass on that there is potential to recover from a disease, if one chooses to take responsibility for it, and to believe that it is possible. Or, in their own words, "In order to make it authentic, essential, and flowing from your deepest truth, you have undertaken to experience what you have with your thyroid gland. You are essentially declaring to the universe, 'I am an alchemist, and this is my way to create, to produce miracles and magical realities in my life, and thereby to bring it into the collective consciousness.' "

Aside from this mental-emotional reinforcement, which personally brought me to tears, I received various types of energetic and frequency inputs that filled the needs in my physical and energetic body and initiated activity on the level of my DNA. On the physical level, I felt currents in my body and something moving really gently in my brain. I received no physical healing to the thyroid gland itself in this treatment. Not because it was impossible—no, this battle could have ended at that gathering. But it didn't.

The channeler asked his "bodiless friends" who were treating me why this was happening, and he was told, "This is hers." They chose not to intervene in healing the thyroid gland because that was what my spirit asked. I got another lesson in the differences between our immediate well-being, our immediate desires, the desire of the temporal soul to "get well already and end this irritating, exhausting, and unending story of hypothyroidism" and the desire of the eternal spirit within us for our greater, supernal good. And that greater good requires the full healing to arrive only at the right time, so that I might learn everything that this disease had come to teach me, without any shortcuts or discounts.

A SMALL BUT GREAT MIRACLE

The month-long break passed and I took the blood test. My TSH had declined in thirty days from 52 to 18.52. A much greater decline than I had dared to ask, dream, or hope for. Wow! What a dramatic decline in only one month, and even crazier if you consider that I did nothing in practice besides practicing the Tibetan exercises and making a plea to God for a sign.

I sent the doctor the amazing results by email. I had to share them with him—after all, he was my partner on this journey. Though I hadn't discussed the matter with him, it was clear that he was thinking about it and that the issue was troubling him. After all, he too was a human being. Most people take their work home with them when they leave the office and doctors do so as well, particularly in cases that are odd or tough or painful or confusing or life-changing. It doesn't end when they leave the hospital or clinic grounds.

My doctor was surprised and delighted to see the positive results. He was not shocked when I told him about my dialogue with God and even wrote back "God is great." He told me to stay off the supplements for now, and to grant myself maximum emotional rest in order to allow my gland to rest, and to ensure I slept at least eight hours every night.

I was surprised because the doctor was telling me exactly what I felt intuitively—no more wars, no more campaigns or unending healing regimens. At this point in my life, I believed my thyroid gland would work itself out and heal fully at the right time. I accepted his recommendation, which matched my intuition, and let go of my preoccupation with my thyroid gland.

A Spiritual Slap

On December 8, I visited a nutrition specialist with whom I had set up an appointment six months in advance, following recommendations that I received from several people whose opinion I valued. She was a naturopath, a channeler, and an astrologer, and specialized in preparing food in accordance with the energetic frequency each type of food had and the way it matched the unique energetic frequency of each individual in order to bring us to perform optimally on every level. After years of reading about dozens of nutritional methods, and reading dozens of books about nutrition, I wanted to finally understand which food matched my specific body physically, energetically and spiritually, while referring, of course, to the story told by my expanded blood tests, which now included many hormones and vitamins.

At the beginning of our meeting, I shared with her the path I had traveled and the healing journey I had undergone and my secret desire to get a 5 in my TSH count so I could put it in this book. She read me the riot act over that desire, and I understood that this desire was creating a polar perception on my part whereas reality had a circular aspect, with no beginning and no ending. I could not define my success or failure on my thyroid gland parameter, and I had sinned against myself by using a black or white measuring system. By defining a TSH measurement of 5 by the end of the month as my benchmark for success or failure, I was projecting a polar structure of ups and downs just as I previously had with my bipolar disorder.

My healing process was constant. My healing occurred daily whenever I spoke to and listened to myself. How I mothered myself, took care of myself, accepted myself, and was close to myself at any given moment was what defined my health. There was no endpoint to the journey of self-healing, only an ongoing process of self-discovery. I learned about myself through my respiratory system, through my digestive system, through my neural and endocrine systems. This process of self-discovery did not, and could not end.

Each of the diseases I had created during my life still existed, dormant; I simply chose now not to recognize them in my life anymore. I had experienced and realized each in turn and together, and I chose to let them go. But none of those diseases were "deleted" as I had asked my doctor to do with my asthma. Not the asthma, not the bulimia, not the bipolar disorder, not my drug addictions, and not my hypothyroidism. That was why, each day anew, I choose myself, stabilize myself, and express myself at any given moment, learning to create my point of balance in order to keep from rising too high or sinking too low.

Balance had to be expressed in my nutrition as well—in the interval between meals (neither eating too fast nor constantly snacking), its temperature (neither too hot nor too cold), its quantities (neither to starve myself nor gorge), and even the environmental conditions (sitting, chewing slowly, and experiencing perfect intimacy with myself).

Of course, I received a detailed list of food that was adapted for my needs and supported the structure of my spiritual, energetic, mental, and physiological personality, as well as a recommendation for a few supplements to support the various deficiencies that my body still had. The essence of the meeting, however, was far more important than the details. The obligation for proof and implementation was mine and mine alone.

An Open Ending

After that foundational meeting, I decided to finally let go of the blood tests. After listening to the message passed along to me by my thyroid gland, I made a choice to remain at 18.52. I would take two follow-up assays a year, but that was that in regard to blood tests.

My self-healing would never end because I was curing myself in each and every moment, as was expressed in every step I took, with my declaration at the beginning of each and every morning that I chose to live in a state of balance, and my choice to act in accordance with this declaration in my thoughts, behavior, actions, the food I put into my mouth, and self-listening. The result no longer really mattered; what mattered was how I took care of myself from that point onward.

Thankfully, there was no turning back from the path I took. This path was maddening, insane, brave, often challenging, sometimes filled with despair, painful, and rocky. It broke me apart and put me back together. I still walk this path in all that relates to balance in the different levels of my reality, and this march will last until the end of my life, but at that point of my life, I was walking from a place of self-acceptance and self-love, while appreciating and feeling compassion for myself.

No, there was no turning back. I was marching forward from the unity of the three elements making up my essence: body, soul, and spirit. This book is my mission. My creation. My expression of love.

SUMMARY

What did I learn about myself from my thyroid gland?

- My body betrayed me because I betrayed myself first.
- The right path for me was a path of balance (body, soul, and spirit) and self-acceptance.
- Every day anew I must accept myself, listen to myself, express myself, and be my own mother.
- Believe, persist, and never give up.
- This book dealing with self-healing was my mission, my destiny.

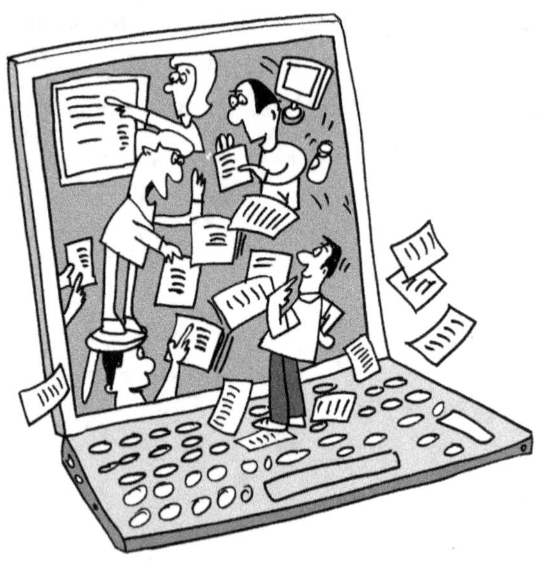

Don't be ashamed to know and don't be ashamed of the information you retrieve from the internet

TIPS, BOOKS, AND MEDITATIONS TO TIDE YOU BY ON YOUR PATH

Congratulations! You have chosen to proactively seek out information about channels and roads that might lead you toward your goal—health. You have chosen to assume responsibility for your health. Be thankful for the fact that you live in an age where the greatest trove of knowledge that has ever existed in the world is at the palm of your hand or on your laptop. That can hardly be taken for granted after thousands of years of ignorance, in which only the rich had access to knowledge and everyone else was an ignorant illiterate who lived in constant existential fear.

You must assume that you need not go to university to study a matter deeply. All you need is a desire to learn more, a healthy curiosity, and persistence. Don't be ashamed to know, and don't be ashamed of the information you retrieve from the internet. It is true that vast amounts of nonsense of all sorts exist online, but treasure troves of knowledge and wisdom are hidden among the grime that can help you increase your confidence in yourself and in the path you have chosen. You must seek and you must want to find.

Stick to YouTube. It has plenty of high-quality materials, surrounded by a great deal of trash of course, but the amount of high-quality materials, which only grows every day and every hour, is more than enough to last you several years. When you expand the search to Google, you risk overload with all sorts of materials and directions that will simply confuse you. You should, of course, use Google when you want to focus and expand your knowledge on a particular point or definition, but in general you should stick to the narrower field of movies, because everything and everyone you will need to know are there. All the experts, all the knowledge, all the stories, all the experiences, all the inspirations. Endless knowledge.

How do you even begin? By optimizing your time. My recommendation is to start with documentaries. Each documentary is the product of the collaborative efforts of the finest minds and many inquiries and cross-referencing of data. For the most part, each documentary concentrates many professionals from many fields. It's all condensed in the documentary. Start with a movie on a subject that interests you, that you want to look into, and from there life will lead you to wherever you are meant to arrive. Everyone is meant to arrive somewhere else, the place that suits them.

Watch online lectures. Listen to lectures given by professionals. Clips fifteen minutes or less are enticing due to their brevity, but represent a bottomless well in which you can easily get lost and lose your focus. A full lecture, on the other hand, has structure, has an introduction, body, and conclusion. The lecturer leads you step-by-step on a path that helps you understand the entire essence of the subject rather than just one small point. It will therefore enlighten you much more than a short clip.

The exceptions to this rule of thumb are **TED Talks.** There is an incredible advantage to the short length of the lectures, since the finest minds have worked very hard to condense all of their knowledge and experience to lectures ten to twenty minutes long in an easy, interesting, enriching, and fascinating way. You can find quite a bit of inspiration there as well.

Seek out and listen to **panels of experts** on subjects that are of interest to you, for two reasons. First, since most experts are time-limited, their arguments will be condensed and they will only express their main points, the bottom line. The other reason is that it enables listening to both sides of the story, making it easier for you to reach a conclusion on what direction feels better or more precise for you. From there, you can move on to explore the preferred path.

Exploit YouTube channels. Someone already did the hard work for you and concentrated a great many materials on the same subject on one easily accessible channel. Enter the channels relevant to you. You will quickly discover them since many of the movies that interest you will already belong to this or that channel, and once you locate it, you will only need to enter that channel and watch the other materials concentrated in it.

Don't be ashamed to operate your internal logic. Don't be ashamed to use your intuition when you watch materials that somewhat contradict the norms and conventions you are familiar with. Having no academic background in the relevant materials is no obstacle, rather it allows you to consider things with an open mind, unlike an academic person who is unwilling to listen to anything contradicting what they have already learned.

Don't dismiss the inner voice drawing you to continue to study the same material, even though your mind is seeking to flee it. People have saved their lives this way. The information you will accumulate is extremely valuable—to you, not to the pharmaceutical companies. Its value is in health. Your health. This same information can improve your life and, for some of you, literally save your life. Purchase it with love.

Below is a partial list of the books that opened my eyes, illuminated my heart, strengthened my soul, increased my courage, shook my world, thrilled me, encouraged me, and helped make me the woman I am today: a healthy and balanced individual who loves herself and others, and dares to connect and fulfill their dreams.[8]

Anticancer: A New Way of Life, Dr. David Servan-Schreiber

Love, Medicine and Miracles: Lessons Learned about Self-Healing from a Surgeon's Experience with Exceptional Patients, Bernie S. Siegel

The Biology of Belief: Unleashing the Power of Consciousness, Matter & Miracles, Dr. Bruce H. Lipton

The China Study, Dr. T. Colin Campbell

---

8   This is only a partial list of the sources I used. It contains only the international books that are easily available in English.

The Path to Love: Spiritual Strategies for Healing, Dr. Deepak Chopra

The Road to Recovery, Dr. Kelly Turner

The Sky's the Limit, Dr. Wayne Dyer

Journey of Souls, Dr. Michael Newton

They Can't Find Anything Wrong! Dr. David Clark

Healing Back Pain, Dr. John E. Sarno

Through Time into Healing, Dr. Brian L. Weiss

How Doctors Think, Dr. Jerome Groopman

Depression-Free for Life, Dr. Gabriel Cousens

You Can Heal Your Life, Louise Hay

Your Health is in Your Hands, Andreas Moritz

The Journey, Brandon Bays

The Recalibration of Humanity: 2013 and Beyond (Kryon), Dr. Carroll Lee

Friendship with God, Neale Donald Walsch

The Five Tibetans, Christopher Kilham

Love is Letting Go of Fear, Gerald G. Jampolsky

The Four Agreements, Miguel Ruiz

A New Earth, Eckhart Tolle

Life After Death, D. Scott Rogo

Proof of Heaven: A Neurosurgeon's Journey Into the Afterlife, Dr. Eben Alexander

Meditations

> *"Imagination is better at finding the obscure than the obvious."*
>
> — Gaston Bachelard

To conclude this chapter, I summarized for you the guided imagery meditations that resonated the most with me in my journey of self-healing, and that I feel have the most significant part in forging the healthy person who I now am. These meditations have not yet concluded their role or left my life. I use them to this day when I carry out "maintenance work" on myself, as need demands, and I teach them in workshops and individually to people I spiritually accompany on journeys of self-healing or personal change.

Their effects on people, both immediate and ongoing, thrills me each time anew. The beauty of this type of work is, to me, the rare combination of the simplicity of the meditations themselves and their effect on all four layers of the individual: physical, mental-emotional, energetic, and spiritual.

When we use guided imagery, we are actually "scamming our mind" and using its supposed weak spot—its inability to distinguish between reality and imagination. If something occurs in our imagination, then it perceives it as occurring in its "virtual reality," and **our body responds accordingly on the biological-biochemical level to this imaginary event, as if it had actually happened.**

This is one reason that athletes and successful businesspeople perform guided-imagination exercises. The see, feel, and experience things before they actually do them. They can see the endpoint of their activity before they even begin it.

That is why guided imagery is so effective in the field of healing the mind and the body as well. People who have recovered from severe diseases or handicaps say that they imagined themselves healthy and functional, and saw it happen in their mind's eye long before they recovered in reality.

Following in their footsteps, and inspired by their success stories, I too made a point of imagining success throughout my long path and I managed to unite the desired reality in my imagination with the material reality in my life. You too are invited to do so. There is nothing to lose besides experiencing a few moments of silence each day and a connection to your true identity and essence.

GENERAL INSTRUCTIONS FOR GUIDED IMAGERY MEDITATION

Every one of us is unique and special. Each of you has a different prism through which you experience and see life, a different personality structure, and a different physical build. Don't be afraid to adapt the guided meditations detailed here to your own unique needs, and to whatever feels right for you.

There are no rules; the only rule is to listen to yourself

and do what feels right for you. There is no "should" or "should not," no "right" or "wrong." You can record yourself on your phone reading this instruction and then listen to it and act upon it during the meditation, or read it and have a friend repeat it, or just memorize it—whatever feels right to you.

There are no set times in which you must perform the meditation, or a given period of time you must perform them for. (It can take five minutes or half an hour, that doesn't really matter.) There is no preferential position or location. You can sit on the floor in the lotus position if you like, or sit on a couch, lie on your bed or on the grass, be indoors or outdoors. Everything is legitimate, and any of the above can be the right way for you. The important thing is to insert this special time into your life.

Intention is more important than the specifics of what you visualize. When you work with guided imagery, everyone sees things differently and for everyone the situations and places that emerge are linked to their unique emotional-mental-associative world. A "walk in nature" will be associated for one individual as a walk on the beach, whereas for a second it might be associated as a walk in a green meadow. For a third, it might be a dark forest. A "ball of light" will be transparent for one individual, opaque for a second, and made of bars of light for a third. If you need to imagine yourself releasing something from within you, your intention during the release itself is a dozen times more important than what you visualize coming out of you, or its color or shape.

Background music: Music is nice as an additional bonus to the meditation, but is really not required. If you feel that soft, gentle music can help you unwind and focus, use it. You can easily find entire tracks of appropriate meditation music on YouTube.

Pay attention to what emerges: Oftentimes, you start with one thing and then suddenly find yourself elsewhere. That's okay. You will reach whatever you are supposed to reach, the places that are waiting for you to reach them. They are more important than whatever the meditation guide says, since they are coming from your internal guide, your supernal self.

Do not be fearful: There is no reason to fear whatever is inside you, whatever you might meet on these imaginary journeys. Whatever emerges will emerge in order to be let go and to be released. The key to self-love, and hence to healing, is to accept yourself and all of your levels, even those that are judged to be less attractive.

It is fine to ask a friend to help guide you through the process, or just be there for you, if you do not want to do it alone, particularly on the last meditation.

Emphasize emotions: The magnetic field that the heart produces is five thousand times stronger than that of the brain. The electric field of the heart is one hundred times stronger than that of the brain. The frequencies generated by our hearts impact the environment around them. If you truly want change, your emotion is most important. Don't be afraid to feel as you visualize what is emerging from your inner depths.

1.   THE SHOUTING HILL: GUIDED IMAGERY

Sit down, be silent, and enter an unwound state with a few slow, deep breaths. Fill your stomach with air and slowly exhale it. You can go through all of your body parts and imagine how each inhalation and exhalation enters and exits that organ, and so on to the next organ. For those of you for whom the order matters, you can start with your feet and move up to your head, whatever suits you.

Feel how your body becomes looser and freer. After you feel relaxed and calm, imagine yourself walking on a path in nature on a pleasant spring day, and even imagine sunrays stroking your face. Notice the hill by the side of the path, and the side path leading up to the top of that hill. You ascend that path to the top of the hill. You know that it is the shouting hill. That is where you can shout out all of your frustrations, nervousness, shame, anxiety, and angst.

Imagine yourself standing on top of the hill and just start screaming, yelling, or shrieking up there—have a wild tantrum if you wish. No one can see you, there is no one and nothing to be ashamed of, and all you need to do is let loose and be cleansed of all your burdens.

Imagine what leaves you as a black cloud, or butterflies, or anything else that comes to mind. The important thing is to imagine your burdens exiting you and leaving you be. Do this until you see in your imagination that there is nothing more to let out, that you are done screaming, and then lie down on the ground. (You can imagine that you are lying on a carpet of flowers.)

Imagine as you relax a great beam of light descending from the heavens straight into your heart—illuminating it, empowering it, healing it—and feel your heart beat with power and with vitality. Let this light flow into the rest of your body and trickle into all the places that have just emptied out this black cloud. See yourself illuminated. Imagine yourself with a big smile on your face. When you feel that you are done, open your eyes and return to the here and now.

One of the advantages of this meditation is that it can be performed in an abbreviated version to carry out a point-specific release of anger or stress. If, for example, you find yourself angry or pissed off in the middle of a workday and you want to get rid of these harsh feelings, enter the restroom for a moment, close your eyes, and imagine yourself on top of the screaming hill. Just imagine the black cloud leaving you while you scream. When you are done, imagine yourself lying on the ground, imagine the white light entering your heart and soothing it. See yourself smiling, and conclude. Immediate relief is guaranteed.

2. *PERSONAL SPACE: GUIDED IMAGERY TO PURGE YOUR-SELF OF FOREIGN ENERGIES AND RELEASE ANGER*

Enter a relaxed state. Once you feel calm and relaxed, imagine that you are surrounded by a one-meter square. It can also be a circle or a rectangle. This square is your personal space and that of your distilled essence. It is clean and white and shiny. Imagine within your space the energies of other people that don't belong to you. You can imagine them as black balls or a black cloud, or anything else your imagination comes up with in any shape or color.

The important thing is to understand that these energies are not yours; they don't belong to you, but to other people. They have invaded your personal space. Someone has angered you or insulted you, and left their energies in your space. That is why you feel as you do. In your distilled form, that is not who you are.

Now all you have to do is get these black spheres out of your space. You can imagine yourself kicking these balls out, blowing them out, blowing them up, or taking a massive vacuum cleaner and sucking them out.

When you see that your space has returned to being white, clean, and pristine, when you have finished cleaning your personal space of everything that is not yours, imagine this great beam of light descending and entering straight into your heart—illuminating it, empowering it, healing it—and feel your heart beat with power and vitality. Let that light wash over the rest of your body, imagine yourself illuminated. Imagine yourself with a great big smile on your face. When you feel that you are done, open your eyes and return to the here and now.

3. *Breaking Down the Wall: Guided Imagery to Open your Heart*

This meditation is intended for those of us who, following past injuries, have surrounded our hearts with a wall in order to keep ourselves from being hurt, in order to keep ourselves from feeling the pain again. This wall, as protective as it may be, often prevents us from feeling the good things in our life and the lives of people nearest to us. Those who feel ready, ripe, and interested to begin feeling more are invited to practice this meditation.

Enter a relaxed state. Once you feel calm and relaxed, imagine that you are looking at yourself. You can imagine yourself from the side or from the viewpoint of your imagined self. Imagine a heart beating in your chest. You can see a thick, tall wall surrounding it. This wall has been there for a long time; it guards you and protects you. You placed it there, but now you are at the point in life when you need to remove it, since it is interfering with your ability to feel everything you want to feel. You are no longer afraid of being hurt because you are strong and independent and no longer need it.

Say in your imagination, "I choose to shatter this wall. I choose to feel," and watch how this wall shatters into thousands of shards. Watch the shards transform themselves in the air into shining fragments of light, and how all this light enters your heart and makes it beat vibrantly.

Imagine yourself going wild with joy and happiness, leaping and screeching like the child you once were. Allow yourself to feel the potential for pure joy within you. See your happiness spread like waves on the sea, like ripples leaving you and continuing to echo onward. When you feel that you are done, smile, open your eyes, and return to the here and now.

4. SPIRITUAL GUIDANCE: GUIDED IMAGERY TO RECEIVE DIRECTION

Enter a relaxed state. Once you feel relaxed and calm, imagine yourself sitting at the beach and watching the waves. State in your imagination that you are requesting a spiritual guide to join you. This guide is sentient energy that has been your companion for all of eternity, knows everything about you, and is interested in passing on information to you that will enable your growth and evolution.

Imagine the person or thing that comes to you. The guide can wear almost any appearance: a sphere of light, an animal, someone familiar, someone strange, or a person from your past. Accept everything you receive gratefully, and thank your guide for coming. Address your guide and ask it a question that has been troubling your mind, a recommendation of a desired means of action or information that can assist you at the present time.

The answer can show up in the form of a word that will suddenly appear in your mind, a memory of an event that has happened to you, an image that will suddenly appear between your eyes, a scene from a movie, a quote from a book, or a sentence one of your loved ones often says. Take what comes, and allow whatever it is to echo within you. If you feel that you require additional precision or clarification, ask for it. The guide is there for you. It does not spoon feed you the answers, but it certainly aims you in the right direction.

When you feel that you are done, thank the guide for coming to your aid and watch it walk away. Then smile, open your eyes, and return to the here and now.

5. *THE INNER CHILD: GUIDED IMAGERY TO DISCOVER BLOCKAGES AND RELEASE CONGEALED PAIN*

This meditation is more complex and is based on the insight that in each and every one of us, regardless of our age, resides an inner child who lives within us and never grows up. This child is you and all that you have experienced. This child is hurt, angry, and scared and is responsible for large portions of your behavior without you even being aware of it. It is an inseparable part of your soul, and it speaks to you in all sorts of languages (chapter 1).

Connecting with your inner child is meaningful and has an immense effect on your life. **This child requires a remedial parent, one that will provide them with all the**

love, attention, and guidance that they never received in the past but that every child needs. This role is yours. You are the parents. There is no one else to get the job done.

If you have children, it will be easier to imagine what you would do if your child would enter a traumatic, painful, or hurtful situation that you yourself experienced as a child. Those who do not have children can imagine the same for a nephew or a child of friends. At first, it is recommended to perform only initial acquaintance meetings, and when it feels right, or when the inner child is ready to cooperate, to bring to the surface traumatic, hurtful, or painful events.

Enter a relaxed state. When you feel relaxed and calm, imagine yourself in a place that feels safe and secure, and ask your inner child to join you. Imagine their age, their clothing. This child does not know you—you are a stranger as far as they are concerned—but you must learn to get them to trust you. Tell the child who you are, that you have come to help, that you love them. Then play with them, embrace them, stroke them, give them compliments, tell them how special they are, do everything that you can imagine to make them feel safe and open up to you.

Remember that this child has spent a great deal of time on their own. They have had a rough time. **Be patient with them. It is important to mention, once again, that the acquaintance phase can take several meetings and cannot be rushed.**

Once you feel that the child is cooperating with you and trusts you, begin to question them gently. What is bothering you? What are you angry about? Who hurt or insulted you? What do you need help with? Listen to them and help them in accordance with their answers and the information that emerges. You can summon someone to your meeting that they are angry with or someone who hurt them (whether an adult or a child) to enable the child to express themselves and their frustration and injury at that person, to help them release the burden, purge the trauma from that incident, and perhaps even forgive the injuring party.

As an adult who has undergone the same experience, you can explain why it is important to talk things over, what your shared experience led to, and how talking it over will help them feel better and smile again. Be their parent, provide them with the support and guidance they require but never received. Hug them and love them, and always make sure to say goodbye after they agreed that you can leave, preferably after you imagined yourselves having fun together, and after you reminded them how much you love them and that you would always be there for them. When you feel that you are done, smile, open your eyes, and return to the here and now.

MESSAGE TO THE READERS

I wrote this book so that you would not need to spend a decade in attempting to heal yourself, as I did. To give you hope that healing yourself from chronic diseases is possible, and give you the inspiration to embark on a journey of self-healing and the practical instructions I was lacking when I embarked on my own journey. We have far more power than we have been led to believe!

Yes, ordinary people who did not go to medical schools have the ability to do what our doctors can't do—achieve complete recovery from chronic illnesses in a way that does not depend on chemicals to balance our systems.